Quintessentials of Dental Practice – 23
Endodontics - 2

Managing Endodontic Failure in Practice

By
Bun San Chong

Editor-in Chief: Nairn H F Wilson
Editor Endodontics: John M Whitworth

Quintessence Publishing Co. Ltd.
London, Berlin, Chicago, Copenhagen, Paris, Milan, Barcelona, Istanbul, São Paulo, Tokyo, New Delhi, Moscow, Prague, Warsaw

British Library Cataloguing in Publication Data

Chong, Bun San
Managing endodontic failure in practice. - (Quintessentials of dental practice; 23. Endodontics; 2)
1. Endodontics
I. Title II. Wilson, Nairn H. F. III. Whitworth, John M.
617.6´342

ISBN 1850970866

ISBN 1-85097-086-6

Foreword

Despite new materials, innovative techniques and a plethora of novel devices, the continuing growth and trend towards more complex forms of endodontics has been accompanied by an increasing need to manage endodontic failures. Such failures pose many, varied challenges which, if successfully overcome, can be both professionally rewarding and a real practice builder.

Managing Endodontic Failures in Practice provides a concise, practical overview of the "when" and "how" to save teeth with an unsatisfactory and often deteriorating endodontic outcome. From diagnosis to the monitoring of successfully re-treated teeth, *Managing Endodontic Failures in Practice* is clearly the work of an endodontist "in the know" and "up to speed" on the latest thinking, developments and techniques.

The valuable experience and enjoyment of reading this book is enhanced by its easy-to read style and the large number of high-quality illustrations included in the text – just as you would expect of a Quintessence publication. Altogether this excellent addition to the *Quintessentials of Dental Practice Series* is a most worthwhile and enlightening volume – ideal continuing professional development for the practitioner visited by patients who present with different forms of endodontic failure.

Nairn Wilson
Editor-in Chief

Preface

With a continuing improvement in oral health and a change in patient attitude, it is no longer acceptable to extract teeth simply because of periapical disease and endodontic failure. Advances in scientific knowledge and technical skills have helped improve the prognosis of treatment, but it may not always lead to the desired healing response in clinical practice. If initial treatment is unsuccessful, practitioners are increasingly expected to possess the necessary knowledge and skills to perform ever more technically demanding procedures to save teeth. The focus on evidence-based treatment has resulted in secondary care providers, such as local oral surgery units, no longer being willing unquestioningly to accept failing endodontic cases for surgery, prior to an attempt having been made to retreat by non-surgical means. The aim of this book is therefore to provide practitioners with an understanding of the biological principles and the practical techniques to handle endodontic failures. To this end, it is hoped that its contents are clear, rational, practical and helpful in dealing with endodontic retreatment situations in everyday clinical practice.

Since careful treatment planning is integral to success, a substantial part of this text is dedicated to case assessment and selection. It is inevitable that there will be some repetition of relevant points. There is a myriad of techniques available to manage the many and diverse retreatment situations. It is impossible to cover them all in this book. Emphasis is placed, however, on principles and techniques relevant to general practice, followed briefly by some insight into more advanced methods. For practical instruction on retreatment techniques, practitioners are encouraged to attend hands-on courses.

Bun San Chong

Acknowledgements

I would like to thank my family, Grace, James and Louisa for their understanding and support and for accepting my periodic absences whilst immersed in writing this book. "Muchas gracias" to Monica for all her help and nursing assistance over the years.

Contents

Chapter 1

Defining Success and Failure

Aim

To review the methods of evaluating the outcome of endodontic treatment, explain the reasons for reported variations of success rate and describe the criteria for success and failure.

Outcome

After studying this chapter, the practitioner should have an understanding of how the concepts of success and failure are defined, the process of evaluating treatment outcome, and the principles of justifying remedial treatment.

Terminology

Endodontic treatment is used as a generic term to cover the whole spectrum of pulp and periapical therapy. Root canal treatment describes a specific procedure for treating the dental pulp when irreversible damage has occurred, or when vitality is compromised by disease or injury. Although there is a distinction between the terms, in this book, endodontic treatment and root canal treatment are used interchangeably, as in common usage.

Introduction

It has been said that there is no such thing as failure, just different degrees of success. There is some truth in this statement and it highlights the difficulties of defining success and failure objectively. Therefore, before looking at how to manage endodontic failure, it is pertinent to consider how failure may be defined.

The Strindberg Concept

The traditional, standard notion of success and failure is based on the stringent criteria encapsulated by the so-called "Strindberg Concept". According to Strindberg (1956) the only satisfactory postoperative outcome, after a predetermined postoperative period, is clinically a symptom-free tooth and radiologically the appearance of a normal periapex. Put simply, "success" is defined as the lack of visible signs of disease while "failure" is defined as the presence of any signs or symptoms indicating disease. Such a concept is very "black and white", with a definite cut-off point.

The "Strindberg Concept" is based exclusively on our knowledge of the disease process and represents an "ideal" concept of disease. It can, however, be perceived as being too dogmatic and inflexible for use in everyday clinical practice.

Methods of Evaluating Treatment Outcome

In theory, there are three methods (clinical, radiological and histological) available to evaluate the results of endodontic treatment (Fig 1-1).

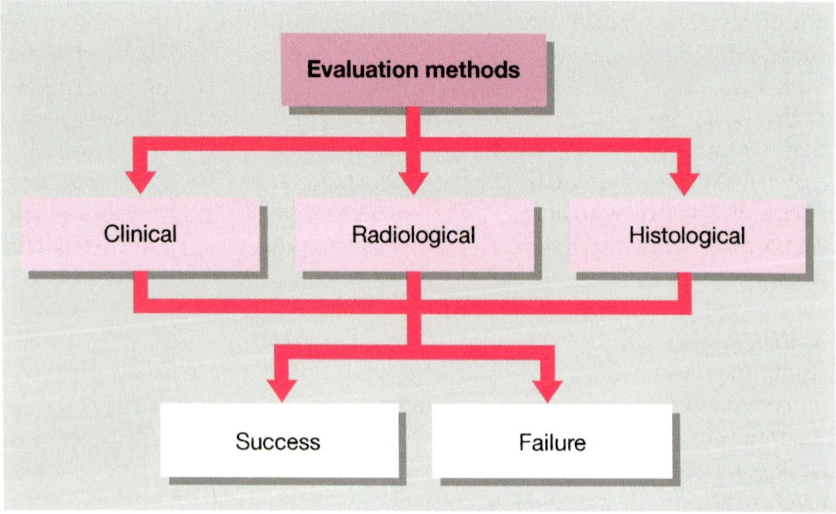

Fig 1-1 Methods of evaluating treatment outcome.

Clinical Evaluation

The patient is questioned about any symptoms experienced, whether the tooth feels normal and is comfortable in function. A clinical examination is then carried out to look for signs of disease such as the presence of:

- a swelling
- a sinus tract (Fig 1-2a) or
- tenderness.

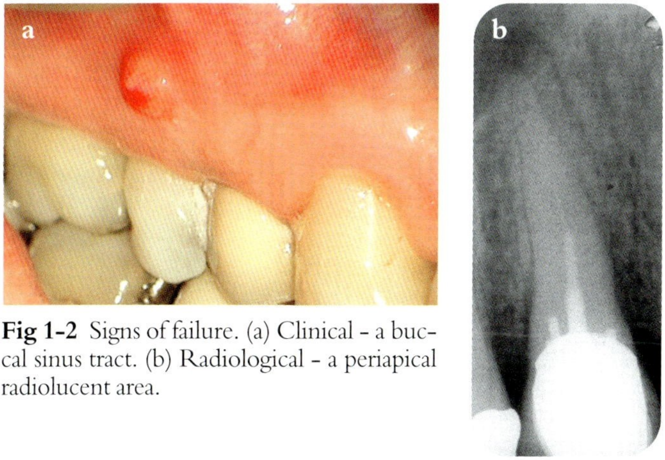

Fig 1-2 Signs of failure. (a) Clinical - a buccal sinus tract. (b) Radiological - a periapical radiolucent area.

An absence of abnormal clinical signs and symptoms is considered indicative of success. There is an element of subjectivity, however, when assessing treatment outcome clinically. Although there is little question if overt signs or symptoms of disease are present, a patient's lack of symptoms may not necessarily mean that the tooth is disease-free and will remain symptom-free. Chronic lesions may have varying presentations, with the patient being unaware of their presence perhaps until, with little warning, alterations in the host/microbial balance transform the dormant lesion into an acute phase; this is something we have all witnessed often.

Radiological Evaluation

Radiographs of the tooth are taken and processed using a standardised technique to ensure a good quality, undistorted image. The radiographs are viewed on a light-box, with magnification and ideally with extraneous light blocked off (Fig 1-3). The following are evaluated:

- quality of the root filling: in particular, its length and density
- periodontal health, including the width of the apical and lateral periodontal ligament space
- presence, location, size and nature of the margin of any radiolucencies (Fig 1-2b) or radiopacities.

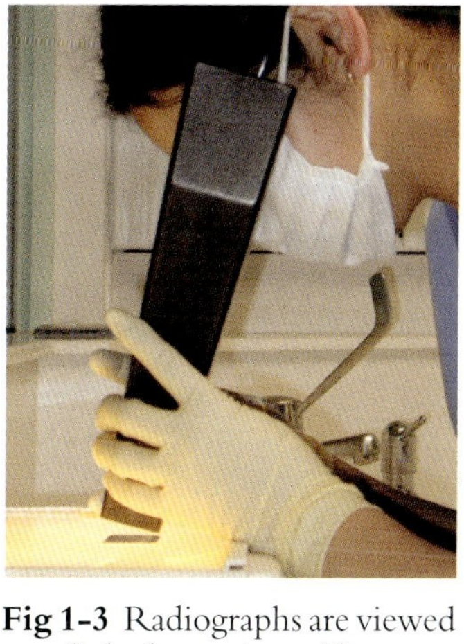

Fig 1-3 Radiographs are viewed on a light-box using a film magnifying cone.

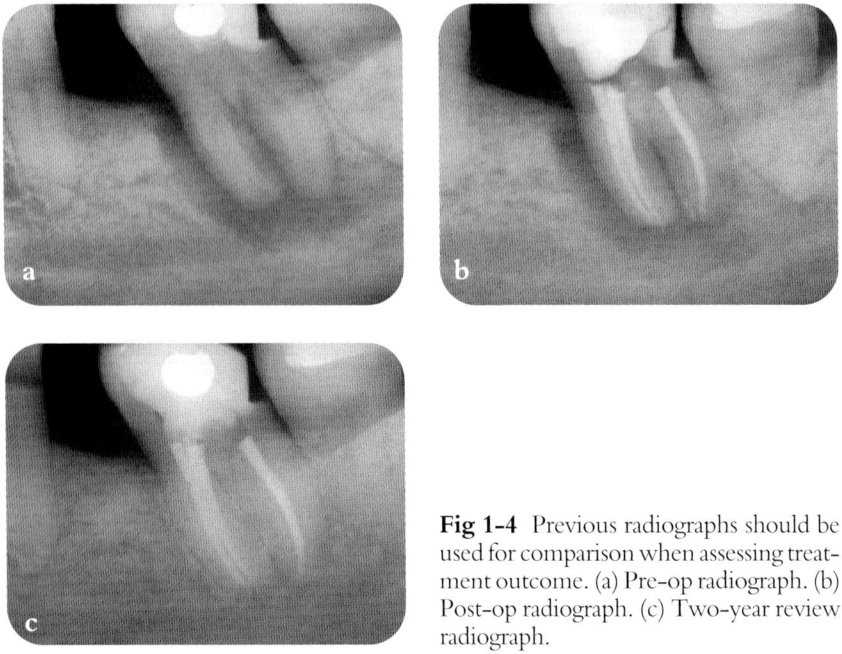

Fig 1-4 Previous radiographs should be used for comparison when assessing treatment outcome. (a) Pre-op radiograph. (b) Post-op radiograph. (c) Two-year review radiograph.

In essence, the task is to detect any features that are not consistent with the radiographic characteristics of healthy periapical tissues. If available, previous radiographs should be used for comparison to ascertain any differences in radiographic appearance with time (Fig 1-4).

A major problem with the radiological assessment of treatment outcome is that:

- not all periapical lesions are detectable - detectability is dependent on the size of the lesion and its location. In addition, a positive radiological finding does not always correspond to the existence of a pathological lesion which needs intervention; for example, healing by scar formation may have occurred (see Chapter 2).

Other difficulties include:

- the need for baseline information to understand follow-up observations and put them in context; there may be a substantial lesion, but it may be reduced in size compared to earlier images
- the problem of inter and intraobserver differences; we are all biased in our judgements and decision-making

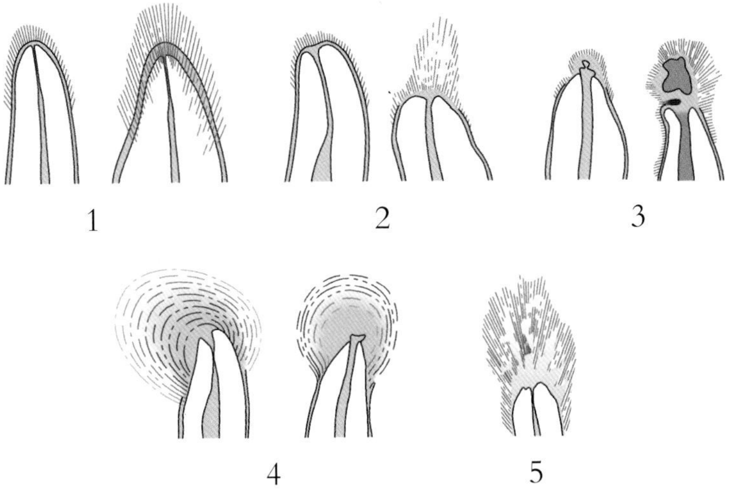

Fig 1-5 The Periapical Index (PAI), a set of five reference visual images denoting either a healthy periapex (score 1) or an increasing extent or severity of apical periodontitis (scores 2-5). (Courtesy of D. Ørstavik.)

- operator bias; if the assessor was responsible for the treatment, it may be difficult to be objective and decisions are likely to be especially loaded. Equally those seeking to intervene may be too condemning in their desire to get on and treat.

Studies have shown that there is relatively poor agreement amongst operators when interpreting radiographs. Although problems with radiological evaluation of treatment outcome cannot be completely eliminated, they can be reduced by:

- formal scoring systems, such as the Periapical Index (PAI), devised to aid radiological assessment of endodontic treatment outcome. In the PAI system (Fig 1-5) a set of five radiographic images denoting either a healthy periapex (score 1) or an increasing extent or severity of apical periodontitis (scores 2-5) is used as a reference when scoring cases
- formal observer calibration; objective observations may be improved with special training
- statistical methods, such as Kappa statistics, an index which compares the agreement against that which might be expected by chance.

Whilst suited to standardised epidemiological surveys, these methods are of limited value in everyday general practice, where an element of judgement and pragmatism based on full understanding of circumstances must prevail. This is not an excuse, however, for uncritical appraisal of failing cases. The monitoring for radiological as well as clinical signs of healing is still important in assessing treatment outcome.

Histological Evaluation

In order to carry out a histological evaluation, surgery is necessary to obtain a block section of the periapex. The block section is processed for histology and examined microscopically. The aim is to determine, at the cellular level, whether there is any evidence of inflammation or other signs of disease at the periapex. The two main problems with the histological assessment of treatment outcome are:

- the need to obtain block sections
- the possibility of artefacts introduced during tissue processing; delicate histological sections may be distorted or damaged.

Purists may consider this method of evaluation the "gold standard", but it is again not a method that is applicable in everyday clinical practice. To biopsy all cases to evaluate healing is clearly unethical and unnecessary, let alone unacceptable to patients.

Reasons for Reported Variations in Success Rates

There are countless reports on the outcome of endodontic treatment and, not surprisingly, differences in reported "success" rates. Whilst it is not the intention of this chapter to review all of them, it is important to say a few words about possible reasons for the apparent lack of consensus.

Case Selection

Studies vary in the teeth included and the degree of technical difficulty in their treatment:

- anterior or posterior teeth
- single or multi-rooted teeth
- a mixture.

There are also:

- varying numbers of subjects
- subjects of different age
- differences in preoperative pulpal and periapical status at the start of treatment.

Treatment Methods

Studies vary greatly in:

- techniques employed for canal preparation, medication and obturation
- materials used
- operator philosophy (e.g. single or multi-visit) and skill.

These variables may be related to operator preference and common approaches contemporaneous at the time of the study. The techniques and materials originally employed may not be relevant to current practice. Operator skill, or the condition under which treatment is delivered cannot be underestimated, epidemiological studies having revealed discrepancies between success rates of endodontic treatment performed in specialist clinics compared with general practice.

Criteria for Evaluation

The difficulties of objective evaluation have already been considered. In research studies, observers should be trained and calibrated, but variations in study methods still remain. These include:

- parameters recorded
- criteria for success and failure
- methods of assessment
- retention of subjects for follow-up in a long-term trial
- observation period
- analysis of results.

Observer Variation

The "human" factor is a recognised variable and can account for reported differences in success and failure studies. As previously mentioned, there are methods including observer training and calibration, and statistical tests of intra and interexaminer reliability to minimise its effects. The effect of the "human" factor and the extent of its influence are, however, difficult to quantify, let alone fully appreciate in studying reports of success and failure.

European Society of Endodontology Guidelines

For practical purposes, practitioners wishing to assess success and failure should adopt guidelines set out by a recognised body of opinion; for example, the European Society of Endodontology (ESE) Guidelines. These guidelines are pragmatic, workable and appropriate for daily use in practice.

According to the ESE guidelines, teeth should be assessed one year after root

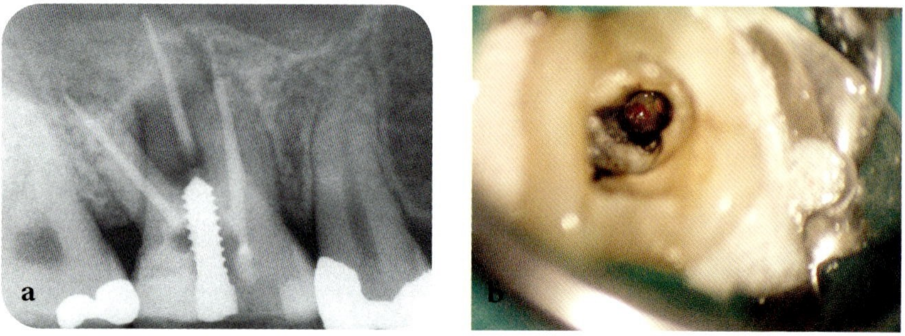

Fig 1-6 Failure due to suspected root perforation. (a) Pre-op radiograph. (b) Perforation confirmed following post removal.

canal treatment and subsequently thereafter as required. The root canal treatment is considered a success or failure dependent on clinical and radiographic findings. In essence, if a root-filled tooth is functional, clinically symptomless and without radiographic evidence of disease, then the root canal treatment is regarded as a success.

Definition of Success

- absence of pain, swelling and other symptoms
- no sinus tract
- no loss of function
- radiographic appearance of a normal periodontal ligament space.

Definition of Failure

- a lesion develops postoperatively or a pre-existing lesion increases in size
- a lesion has remained the same or only diminished in size during a four-year assessment period
- symptoms and radiographic findings are contradictory
- there are signs of continuing root resorption or hypercementosis.

Whilst many teeth respond "successfully" to root canal treatment, many probably fall into an "undecided" category; not really in need of intervention now, but not a complete "success" in these terms either. The various considerations to take into account when deciding on intervention are covered in Chapter 3.

Ideally, all root canal treated teeth should be monitored clinically and radiographically. Regardless of the technical quality, root treated teeth can

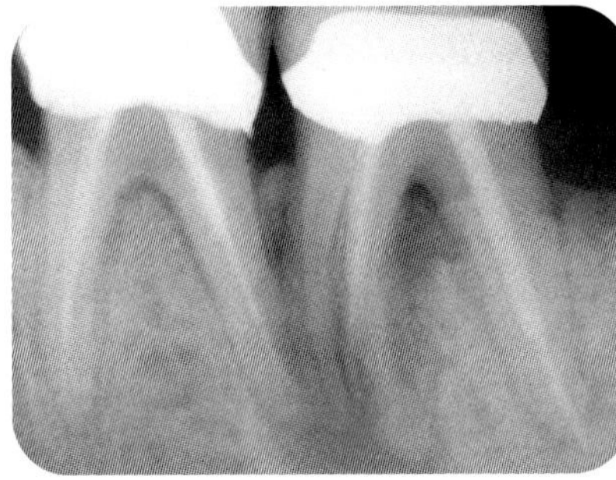

Fig 1-8 Failure due to root fracture.

become failures following changes in circumstances; for example, subsequent to loss of a coronal restoration, accidental root perforation during post space preparation (Fig 1-6) or root fracture (Fig 1-7). Monitoring is also important because failures are not infrequent. Indeed, failures can be a sizeable problem. If root canal treatment is considered to have a success rate of around 90%, then for every ten cases there is one failure. In England and Wales alone, the number of patients undergoing root canal treatment on the National Health Service exceeds one million a year. A 10% failure rate will result in over 100,000 treatment failures each year - a very large number of failed cases by any reckoning. It is a clinical challenge, let alone the expectation of our patients, to try and save some of these teeth. Therefore, practitioners need to know and develop skills to manage endodontic failures.

Conclusions

- Treatment outcome may be evaluated clinically, radiologically or histologically.
- Success and failure may be defined in many ways, ranging from being empirically derived to more formal, stringent criterion-based assessments.
- Variations in assessment methods results in differences in the reported success rates of endodontic treatment.
- For practical purposes, a widely accepted definition of success and failure should be adopted for everyday use in clinical practice.
- The definition of endodontic failure may not necessarily demand immediate remedial intervention; there are various considerations to take into account.

Intraradicular infection

Persistent intraradicular infection occurs most frequently when the original treatment falls short of acceptable technical standards (Fig 2-1a). Cross-sectional surveys from various countries have revealed that, on average, 30% of endodontically treated teeth are associated with periapical radiolucencies and there is a positive correlation with poor technical quality of the root filling. Unfortunately, radiographs, typically taken in a buccolingual direction, rarely tell the whole story. Apparently well-treated cases may have, for example, obvious deficiencies in the third dimension or missed canals (Fig 2-2). Failures associated with technical deficiencies are usually amenable to non-surgical retreatment (Fig 2-1b).

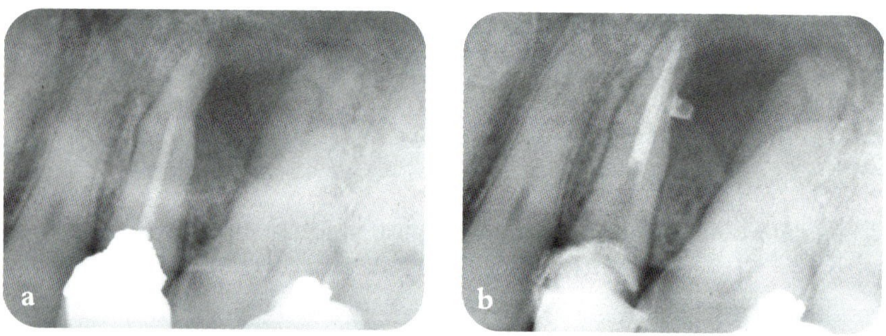

Fig 2-1 Persistent intraradicular infection. (a) Poor technical quality root filling. (b) Managed by non-surgical retreatment.

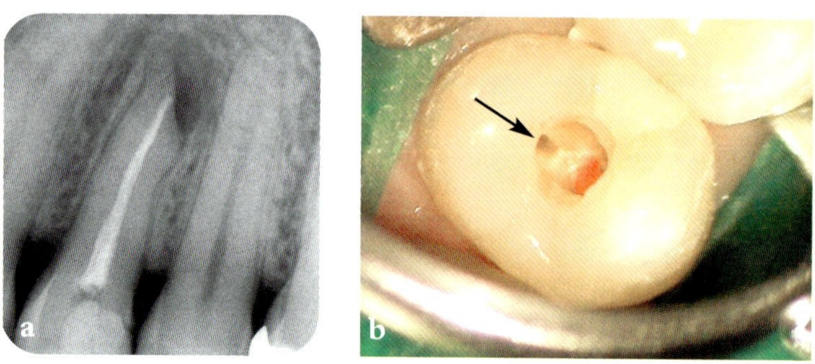

Fig 2-2 Do not go by looks alone! (a) An apparently well root filled tooth. (b) The missed, untreated palatal canal (arrowed).

Extraradicular infection

Failures in cases in which a high technical standard of treatment has been attained are more challenging to handle and resolve. Often, it is difficult to identify the reason for this type of failure. Studies have suggested that therapy-resistant cases may be associated with some form of extraradicular recalcitrant infection - an established infection colonising the external root face, forming a biofilm and persisting in periapical tissues. Inaccessible and unresponsive to conventional root canal treatment, the infection also resists the efforts of the host defences. *Actinomyces israelii* (Fig 2-3) and *Propionibacterium propionicum* have been reported to be associated with extraradicular infections.

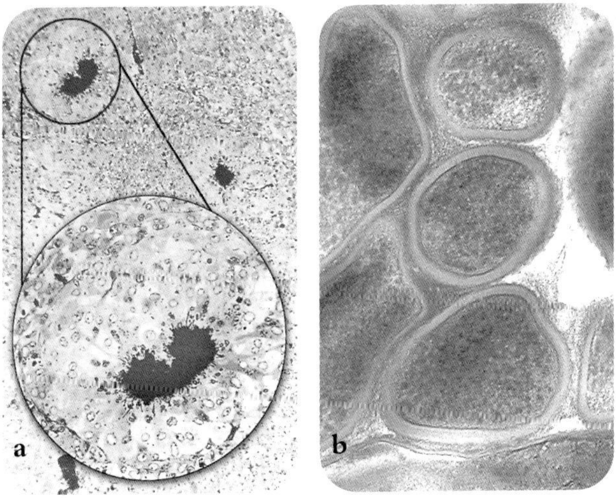

Fig 2-3 *A. israelii.* (a) Light microscope view showing several colonies, magnified inset shows typical "ray fungus" appearance of actinomycosis. (b) Electron microscope view of ultrastructure, Gram-positive cell walls surrounded by extracellular matrix. (Courtesy of D. Figdor.)

Typically, a radical approach, including a combination of surgical and non-surgical retreatment, may be required to deal with therapy-resistant cases (Fig 2-4). Even then, not all affected teeth can be saved. It should be noted, however, that non-surgical retreatment is almost always justified as a first-line approach for managing failures associated with apparently well root treated teeth (see Chapter 3 and Fig 2-5).

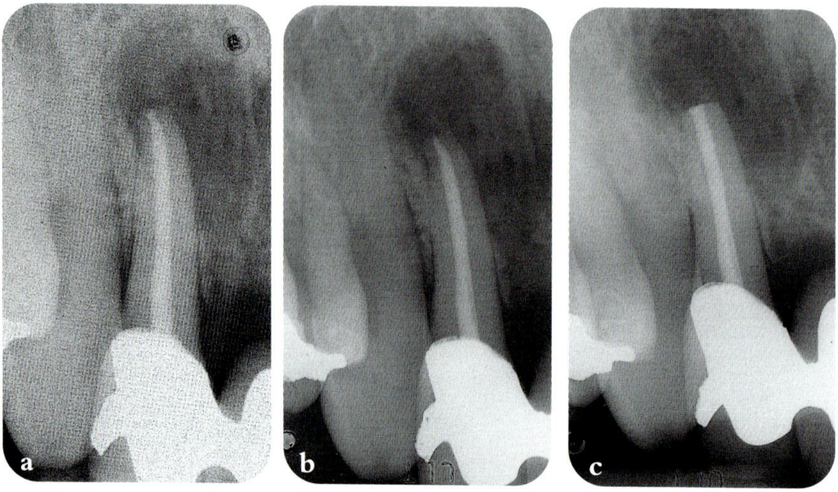

Fig 2-4 Failure due to extraradicular infection. (a) Initial root canal treatment. (b) Six-month review, the periapical radiolucency increased in size. (c) Immediately following combined non-surgical and surgical retreatment. Biopsy report revealed infection caused by *A. israelii*.

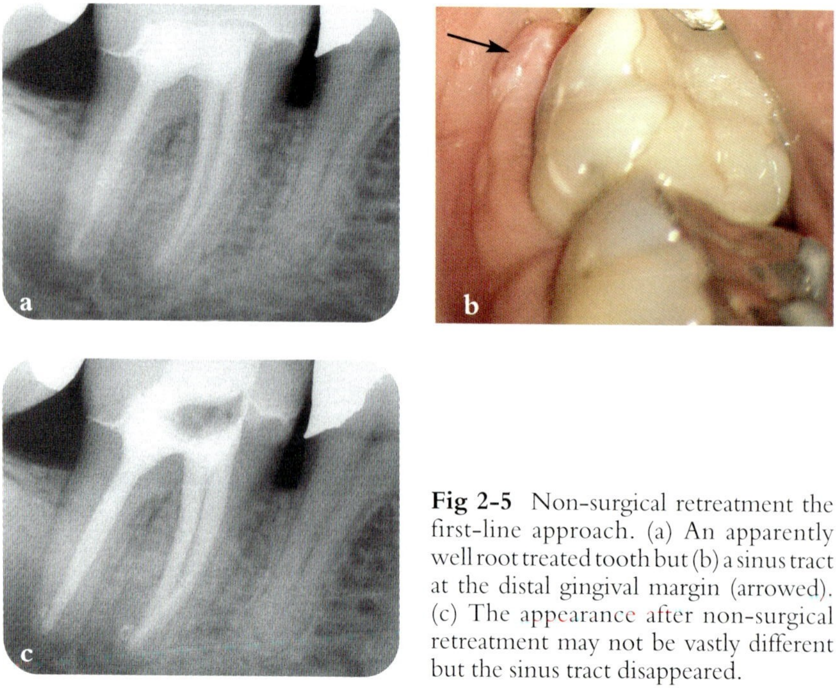

Fig 2-5 Non-surgical retreatment the first-line approach. (a) An apparently well root treated tooth but (b) a sinus tract at the distal gingival margin (arrowed). (c) The appearance after non-surgical retreatment may not be vastly different but the sinus tract disappeared.

Cysts

Any periapical lesion ≥ 1 cm in diameter with well-demarcated margins is usually considered likely to be a cyst. Radicular cysts which are inflammatory in origin can be divided into (Fig 2-6):

- Apical pocket cysts - in which the epithelial-lined cystic cavity is in communication with the root canal system.
- Apical true cysts - in which the cystic cavity is completely enclosed in epithelial lining, separated and has no communication with the root canal system.

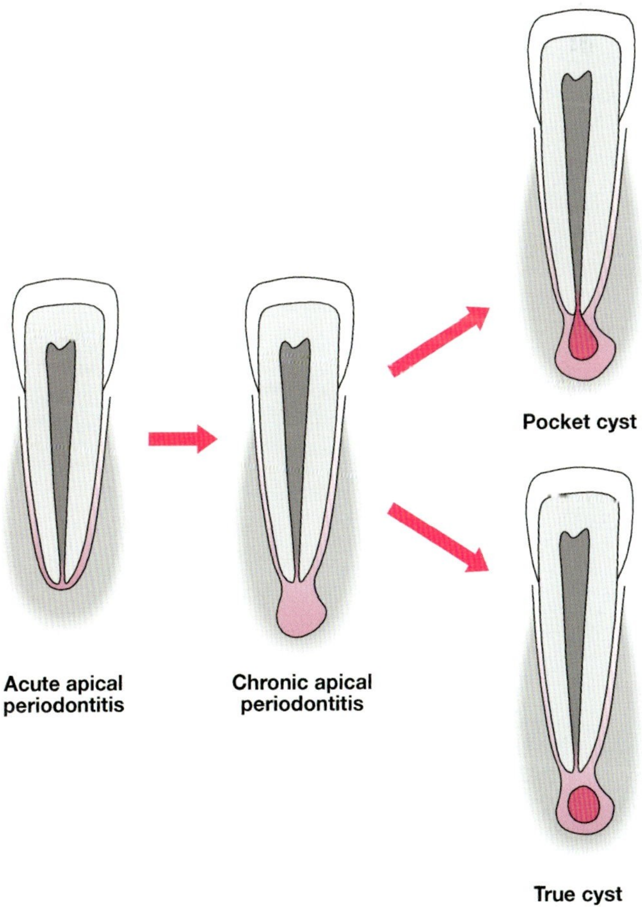

Fig 2-6 Development of the two types of radicular cysts.

With an apical pocket cyst, healing will usually occur following successful non-surgical retreatment. A true cyst, on the other hand, in which the tissue dynamics are self-sustaining, is unlikely to resolve with non-surgical retreatment. Surgery is usually indicated to enucleate an apical true cyst but, unfortunately, it is impossible to differentiate between the two types of cysts before treatment.

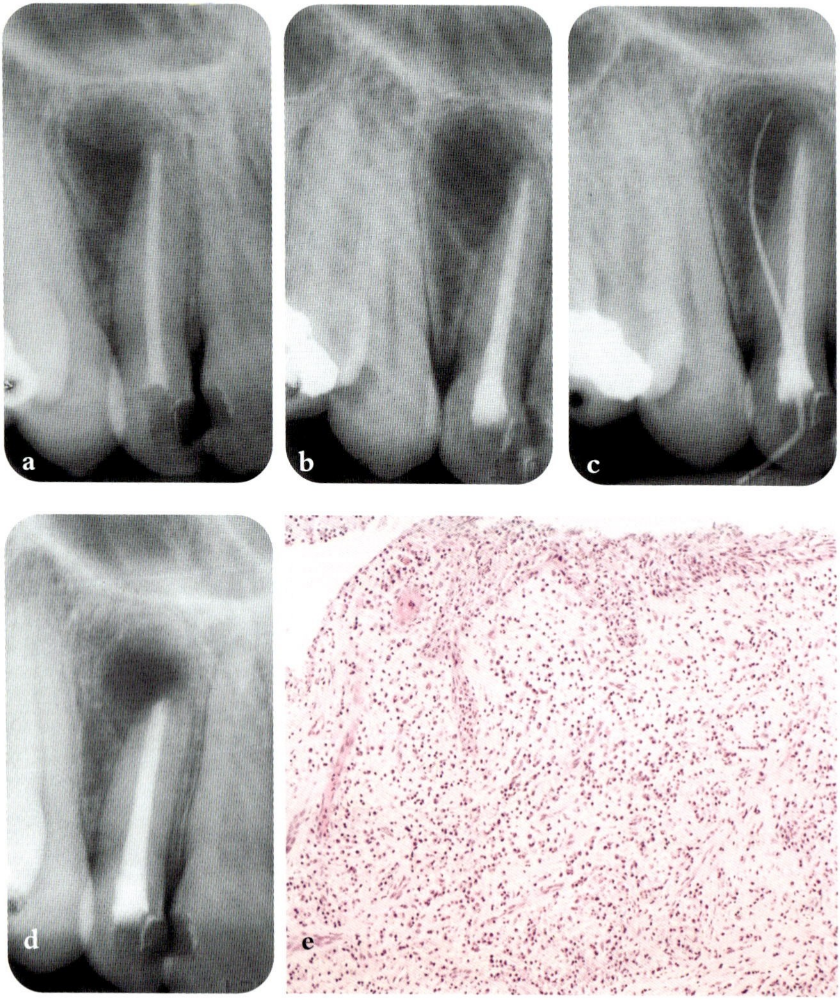

Fig 2-7 An apical true cyst. (a) Periapical radiolucency despite an adequate root filling. (b) Non-surgical retreatment performed. (c) Failure: a sinus tract appeared, traced with gutta percha cone. (d) Surgical retreatment performed. (e) Histological section of biopsy material confirmed an epithelial-lined true cyst.

Therefore, even if an apical true cyst is suspected, non-surgical retreatment should still be carried out in the first instance and the outcome monitored before a decision is made on the necessity for surgery (Fig 2-7).

Foreign Body Reaction

A giant cell reaction, due to the inadvertent introduction of foreign bodies, including food particles and endodontic materials (Fig 2-8), into the periapex, may result in endodontic failure. Typically, the culprit is cellulose from:

- paper points
- cotton wool
- food debris.

In the case of food particles, the teeth involved are usually broken down or lacking a coronal restoration, and the root canal has become exposed, allowing the ingress of foreign material.

Endodontic materials in the periapex may evoke a foreign body reaction, in response to:

- the root filling material itself
- contaminants in the root filling material such as talc.

In these cases, if the periapical radiolucency persists and the foreign body reaction is limited, no attention is required. If the tooth is giving rise to symptoms, however, then treatment is indicated. Failures of this type are usually only responsive to surgical retreatment (Fig 2-9) since retrieval of extruded material is difficult by the orthograde route.

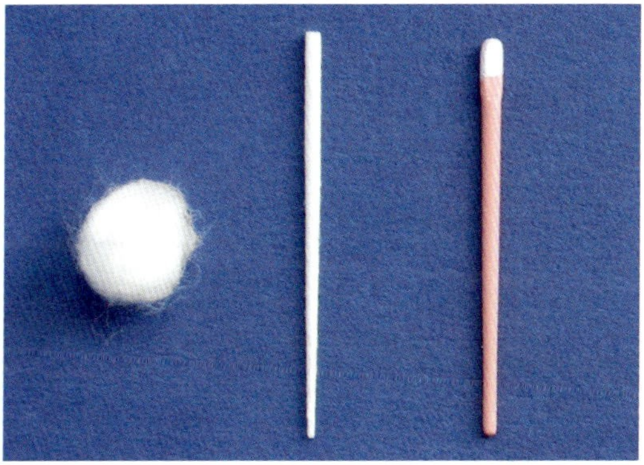

Fig 2-8 Root filling materials or cellulose fibres from cotton wool or paper points in the periapex may evoke a foreign body reaction.

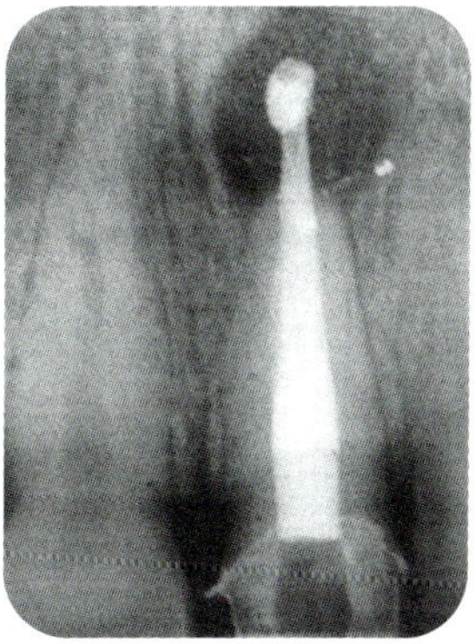

Fig 2-9 Overextended root filling requiring surgical retreatment.

Fibrous Healing

Occasionally, a periapical radiolucency is only reduced in size or in certain cases remains the same size following endodontic treatment. If the width of the periodontal ligament space is within normal limits, the lamina dura is intact, and there are no untoward clinical findings, this may indicate fibrous healing or healing by scar formation.

Fibrous healing is a feature most often associated with periapical surgery. Since the bone adjacent to a periapical lesion is removed during surgery, the periapical radiolucency initially looks more marked. The dynamics of post-surgical healing can result in a variable and irregular radiolucency. If fibrous healing with scar tissue formation occurs, the trabecular bone pattern radiating from the centre will manifest as a reduced but incompletely resolved radiolucency (Fig 2-10).

A persistent radiolucency may also be seen with healed lesions following non-surgical endodontic treatment. This happens if both buccal and lingual or palatal cortical bone plates were perforated by the original infection or inflammation and are not reformed.

In surgical endodontics, guided tissue regeneration techniques (see Chapter 8) have been applied to encourage complete bone reformation, in particular where a large periapical lesion involving buccal and lingual or palatal cortical plates existed.

Infection-free fibrous healing or healing by scar formation is not technically a failure. Unfortunately, without the benefit of histological analysis, it is impos-

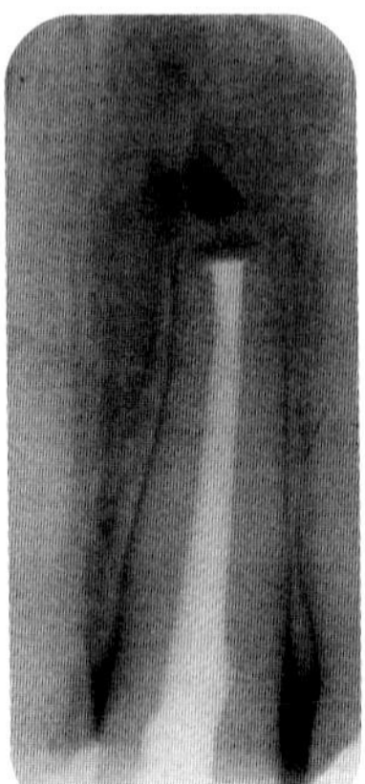

Fig 2-10 Fibrous healing postsurgery, characteristic appearance of a variable and irregular residual radiolucency. (Reproduced with permission from Chong et al. 2003, Int Endod J, Blackwell Publishing, Oxford.)

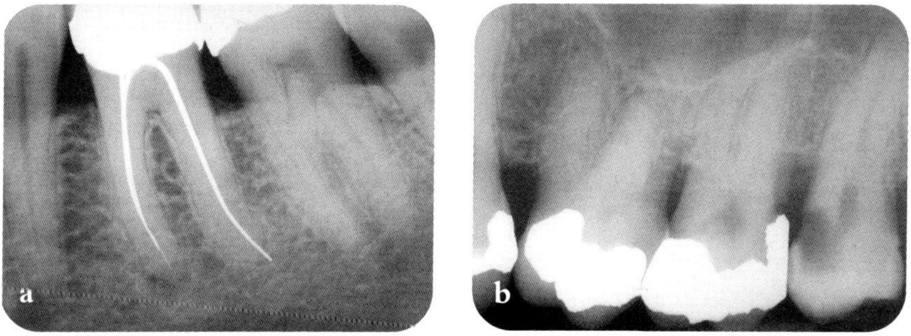

Fig 2-11 Potential misdiagnosis. (a) Is the root filling in the mandibular first molar failing? (b) The culprit is the maxillary third molar!

sible to be certain of the nature of the periapical radiolucency. The desire to intervene in an obviously symptom-free tooth should be carefully considered.

Misdiagnosis

It may be obvious, but a percentage of recorded failures may be misdiagnoses (Fig 2-11). The wrong tooth may have been treated or the cause of the original problem may have been misdiagnosed. Again, radiographs, typically taken in a buccolingual direction, may not reveal the full complexity of the root canal system, let alone the presence of any additional roots. Unless correctly diagnosed, inappropriate and inadequate treatment may have been provided.

Another example is the so-called "cracked tooth". If an incomplete fracture escaped notice, then irrespective of a technically well-performed root filling, and particularly if there is no protective coronal restoration, the crack will propagate further allowing coronal leakage, leading to failure. Even if the crack is diagnosed, sometimes it may be more extensive than suspected. After the root canal treatment, and despite the placement of a coronal restoration to splint the tooth together, further crack propagation continues and ultimately catastrophic failure occurs (Fig 2-12).

Conclusions

- In cases in which the desired healing response has not occurred following endodontic treatment, non-surgical or possibly surgical retreatment should be considered rather than condemning the tooth to extraction.
- There are a number of causes of endodontic failure; the commonest are persistence of the original infection, or new infection due to coronal leakage, especially where there is a poor-technical-quality root filling.

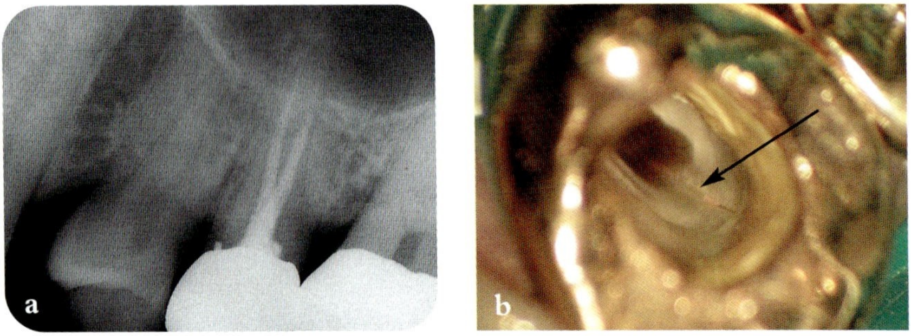

Fig 2-12 Failure due to a cracked root. (a) Tooth with an adequate root filling and a gold crown. (b) Further investigation revealed the presence of a crack (arrowed).

- Persistent infection is usually, though not always, associated with poor-quality treatment.
- Although a root filling may look technically satisfactory, deficiencies may be present, often only discovered when the tooth is retreated.
- Even if the appearance of the root filling is not improved, non-surgical retreatment can improve the internal environment and promote health, and is almost always justified as the first-line approach for managing endodontic failures.
- Therapy-resistant cases may be due to the presence of extraradicular infection, which may not be amenable to conventional non-surgical retreatment. Such lesions can only be identified after carefully conducted retreatment.

Further Reading

Chong BS, Pitt Ford TR, Hudson MB. A prospective clinical study of Mineral Trioxide Aggregate and IRM when used as root-end filling materials in endodontic surgery. Int Endod J 2003;36:520-526.

Figdor D. Microbial aetiology of endodontic treatment failure and pathogenic properties of selected species. Umeå University, Umeå: Sweden, Odontological Dissertations No. 79, 2002.

Nair PNR. New perspectives on radicular cysts: do they heal. Int Endod J 1998;31:155-160.

Nair PNR. Apical periodontitis: a dynamic encounter between root canal infection and host response. Periodontology 2000 1997;13:121-148.

Noiri Y, Ehara A, Kawahara T, et al. Participation of bacterial biofilms in refractory and chronic periapical periodontitis. J Endod 2002;28:679-683.

Siqueira Jr JF. Aetiology of root canal treatment failure: why well-treated teeth can fail. Int Endod J 2001;34:1-10.

Siqueira Jr JF. Endodontic infections: concepts, paradigms, and perspectives. Oral Surg Oral Med Oral Pathol Oral Radiol Endod 2002;94:281-293.

Sunde PT, Olsen I, Debelian GJ, Tronstad L. Microbiota of periapical lesions refractory to endodontic therapy. J Endod 2002;28:304-310.

Takahashi K. Microbiological, pathological, inflammatory, immunological and molecular biological aspects of periradicular disease. Int Endod J 1998;31:311-325.

Chapter 3
The Decision-Making Process

Aim

To review the factors influencing rational decision-making, when to treat and when not to treat failed endodontic cases.

Outcome

At the end of this chapter, the practitioner should be able to appreciate the many factors influencing decision-making, decide on the necessity, timing and preference for retreatment.

Introduction

"Decisions, decisions, decisions", from deciding that a case has failed, to deciding the cause of failure, and deciding if any and what action is needed, a major part of managing endodontic failures revolves around the decision-making process (Fig 3-1).

Decision-Making

Clinical decision-making is a complex task, often characterised as an informal intuitive process and regarded more as an art than a science. Arguments can often be made in both directions. Decision-making is about balancing risks: to intervene or watch and wait, to manage surgically or non-surgically. Finding the right balance is often imprecise but the intention should always be to avoid:

- undertreatment - leaving infection untreated and the patient at risk of local or systemic morbidity
- overtreatment - treating a healthy tooth unnecessarily or where, on balance, the patient has chosen to live with a chronic, symptom-free lesion for the time being.

The decision-making process starts when the patient and dentist first meet. Data collection centres on history taking, followed by a clinical

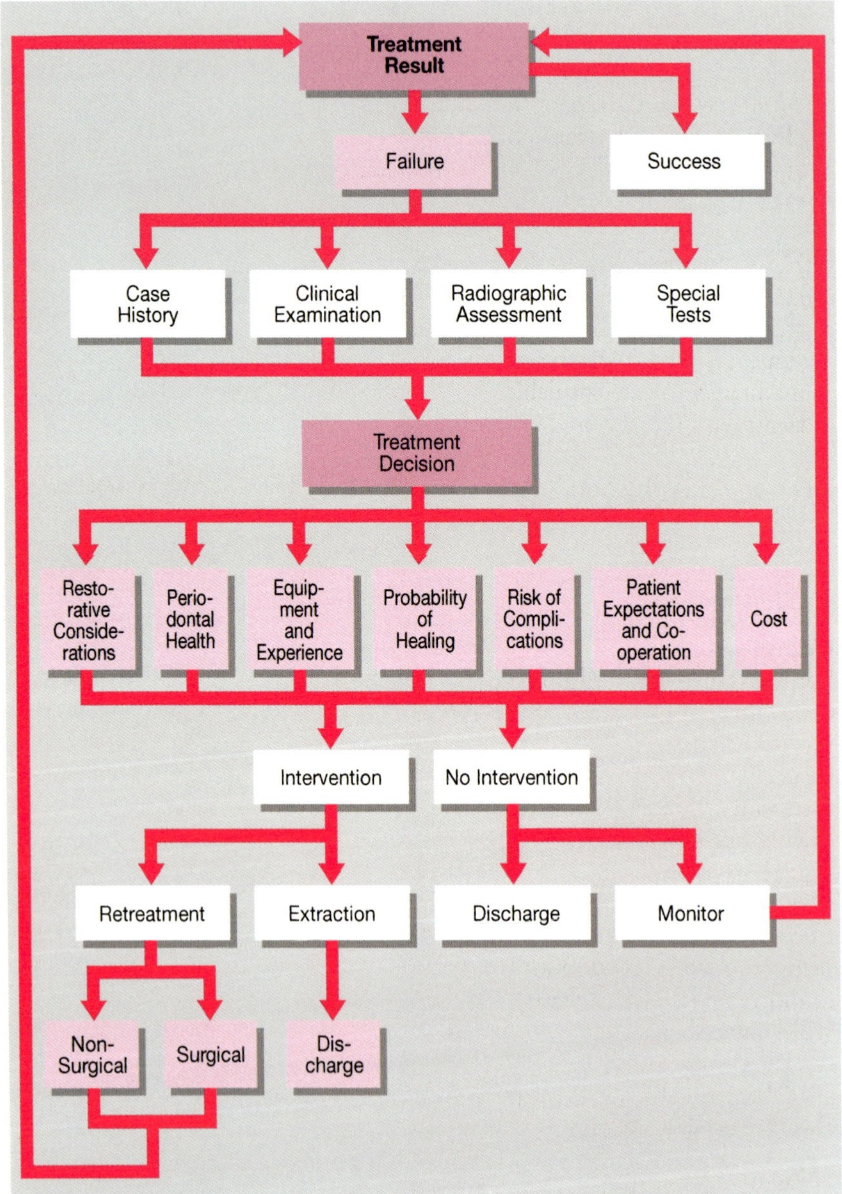

Fig 3–1 The complicated decision-making process when managing endodontic failure.

examination and special tests. Armed with the necessary information, the clinician, relying on knowledge of the presentation of different diseases, makes a diagnosis. Then, a decision on treatment is made based on the:

- clinician's knowledge of the prognosis of the disease
- effect of different treatment options
- anticipated outcome
- patient's personal preference.

Other factors will also come into play, affecting rational decision-making, these include:

- attitudes of both the clinician and patient
- values: in particular, the cost/benefit to the patient
- financial resources available, including the funding of alternative forms of treatment.

It is considered important to review the information feeding into the decision-making process.

Case Selection

Case History

Some patients are well informed, motivated and have a good recollection about any previous endodontic treatment. In contrast, others are poorly motivated and may not even realise that the tooth in question has been previously root treated. A comprehensive history of the previous treatment of the tooth, ideally in chronological order, is helpful and should cover the following questions:

WHAT endodontic treatment has previously been provided?
Endodontic therapy includes root canal treatment, pulp capping, pulpotomy and surgical endodontics. Sometimes a tooth may have had more than one of these procedures performed. Details of previous treatment will enable an assessment as to the feasibility of retreatment or whether the tooth has indeed come to the end of the road. Dental records, when available, should be consulted as patients may often not be fully informed about previous treatment.

WHY was the previous treatment required?
Information on the original complaint which led to endodontic treatment provides an indication of the pretreatment status of the pulp and periapex. The history of the management of the tooth will also help explain

any presenting findings – for example, root resorption – and provide an indication of prognosis. In general, the success rate for the retreatment of teeth with a previously vital pulp is higher than in non-vital cases. Likewise, the success rate for the retreatment of teeth with obstructed root canals is dependent on the preoperative pulpal status and the presence or absence of a periapical radiolucency.

WHEN was treatment carried out?
Knowing how long ago the original treatment was carried out may provide clues about techniques or filling materials that may have been used. Materials and techniques which were once fashionable may now be considered obsolete.

By WHOM was the treatment carried out?
Standards of treatment can vary from one dentist to another. The level of expertise, time and financial constraints may have dictated the use of less than ideal techniques and materials; notwithstanding, all practitioners are expected to provide high standards of treatment.

WHERE was the treatment carried out?
Endodontic techniques practised and materials used vary from country to country and with different treatment philosophies. For example, paste-type root canal filling materials may still be popular in some countries. International air travel means patients are increasingly more mobile; they may have had treatment carried out in another continent. It is therefore relevant to know where treatment was performed and have an appreciation of international variations in endodontic treatment.

Clinical Examination

Extraoral examination
The patient's face and neck are examined for signs of:

- swelling (Fig 3-2a)
- tenderness
- asymmetry
- sinus tracts (Fig 3-2b)
- lymphadenopathy, specifically swelling or tenderness of the cervicofacial lymph nodes.

The extent of the patient's mouth opening should also be evaluated. Access and visibility often dictate the ease of performing retreatment. Limited access may be the reason why the original root treatment was less than satisfactory. Access for retreatment is generally considered inadequate if a patient's mouth opening is less than two-fingers' breadth but every case should be considered individually. It is difficult, for example, to access a molar tooth which is at the back of a very small mouth. By contrast, surgical retreatment of anterior teeth, even if access is limited, may be achievable with the patient's mouth closed for most of the procedure.

Intraoral examination

The dental tissues surrounding the tooth and its neighbours are inspected visually and palpated to detect the presence of any:

- swelling (Fig 3-2c)
- sinus tract
- tenderness.

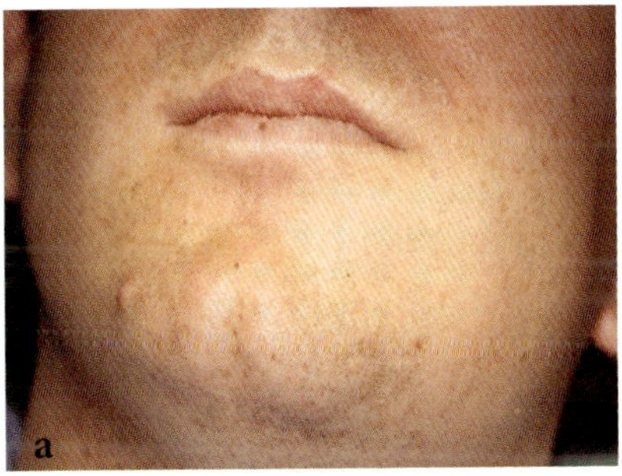

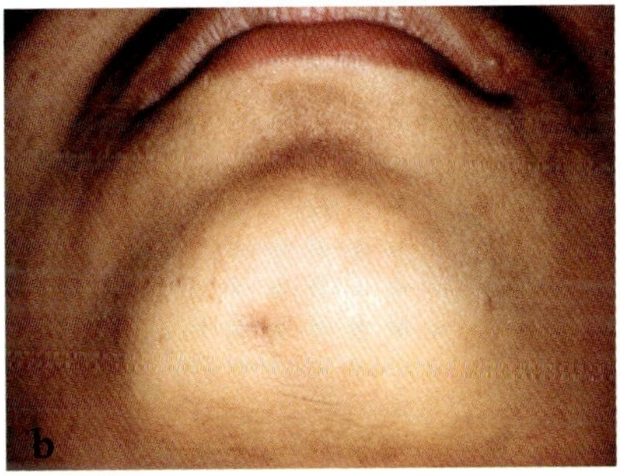

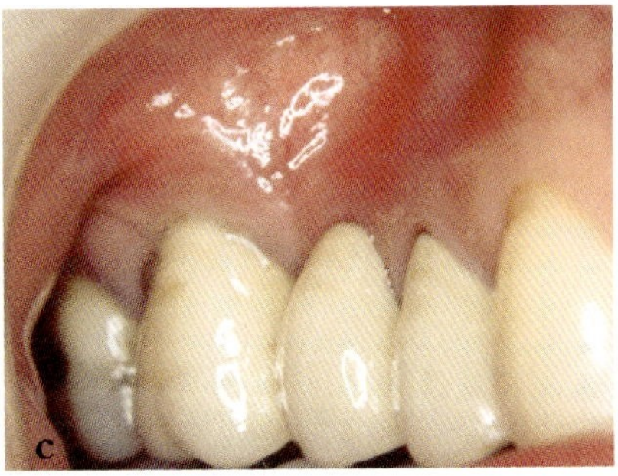

Fig 3-2 Clinical examination may reveal: (a) facial swelling; (b) remnant of an extraoral sinus tract; (c) an intraoral buccal swelling.

If present, a sinus tract should be explored by inserting a gutta percha cone and taking a radiograph to track the source of the infection. It must not be assumed that a sinus tract in proximity to a tooth is evidence of that tooth being the culprit. Infections tend to track through tissues following the path of least resistance, so the source may be some distance from a sinus opening.

The tooth is also checked for:
- quality and quantity of periodontal bony support
- mobility
- tenderness to pressure
- cracks
- colour, compared with adjacent teeth.

To determine if there is any tenderness or mobility, the tooth is percussed or assessed by means of finger pressure. Tooth mobility, if present, should be graded and recorded.

The presence of cracks may be determined by carrying out a "bite test"; this consists of biting on any object which produces a wedging effect and a painful response, which is relieved by releasing the bite. This test is, however, of limited reliability when teeth have already been root treated. In such cases, transillumination (Fig 3-3) may prove useful. If a crack is present, the light transmission will be altered, rendering the crack visible. Magnification, if available, may further help crack detection.

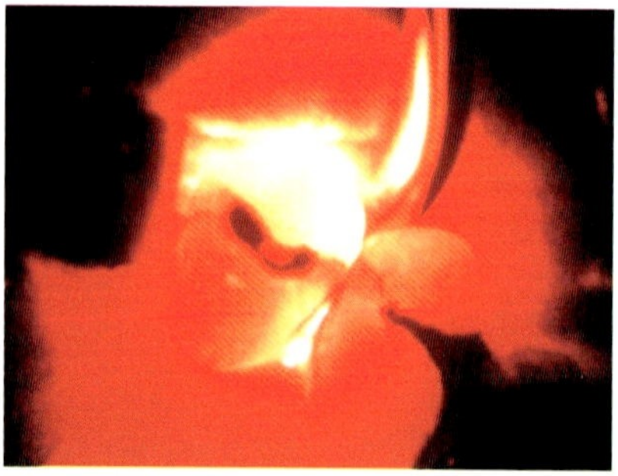

Fig 3-3 Crack detection by transillumination.

Radiographic Assessment

Good-quality radiographs are an essential part of the assessment of previously root treated teeth. Guidelines on quality assurance in dental radiology should be followed to optimise diagnostic information whilst limiting the radiation

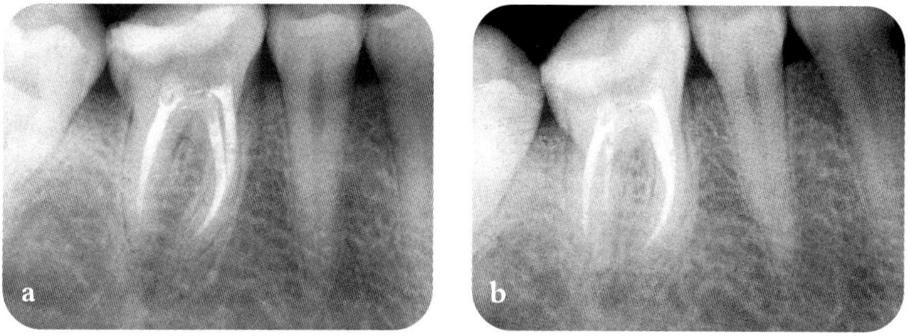

Fig 3-4 What you see and what you don't? (a) Radiograph showing an adequate root filling. (b) A second radiograph, taken at a different angle, revealed inadequacies and a second distal root.

doses to as low a level as reasonably practicable. Radiographs should be taken by the paralleling technique using beam-aiming devices. Additional angled radiographs may be required to build a three-dimensional (3D) understanding of the case (Fig 3-4). As mentioned in Chapter 2, the quality of the radiographic images is dependent on proper handling, processing and viewing of the films.

Clear, undistorted radiographs with good contrast (Fig 3-5) will help determine the:

- quality of the previous root filling and existing coronal restoration
- type of root filling material present
- occurrence of any procedural errors
- possible cause of failure
- likelihood of success in retreating a tooth.

It should also reveal the:

- number of roots and canals present
- root and canal shape and curvature
- other relevant information on the previous root filling.

The quality of the coronal restoration, width of the periodontal ligament space, and the presence, location, size and nature of the margin of any radiolucencies or radiopacities should all be noted.

If available, previous radiographs should be used for comparison to determine whether a periapical lesion is enlarging, remaining the same size or healing

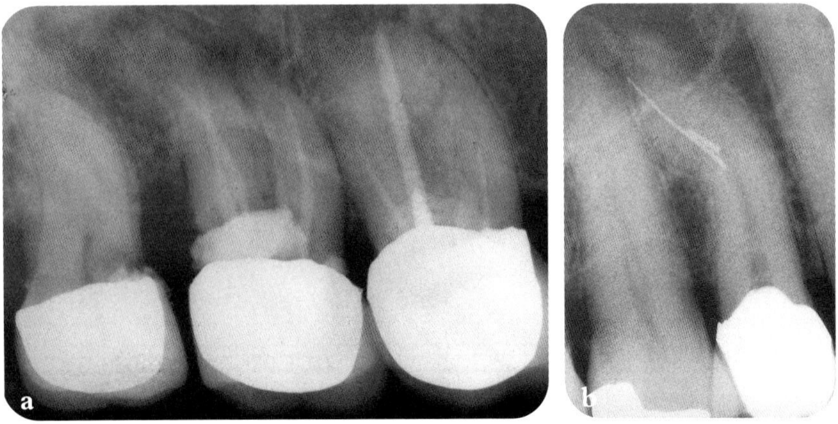

Fig 3-5 Quality radiographs are essential; they reveal: (a) inadequate root fillings in both the first and second molars, caries under the crown in the second and third molars and possible furcal perforation in the second molar and (b) a complicated root canal morphology and two retained instruments in the first premolar.

slowly. If a lesion has remained the same size radiographically or remained relatively large despite some reduction in size, the previous treatment cannot be considered a success but neither is it a clear failure. In this situation, according to ESE guidelines (see Chapter 1), it is advisable to review the case until the lesion has resolved, or for a period of up to four years. After this time the root canal treatment may be considered a failure if total repair has not occurred (Fig 3-6). What remedial action is then taken will depend on the presence of any other signs and symptoms, and following detailed dialogue with the patient.

Restorative Considerations

The state of the tooth and the condition of any existing restorations, including the presence of caries have bearings on selection for retreatment. Caries and defective restorations must be removed to assess the restorability of the tooth (Fig 3-7). There must be sufficient tooth structure to enable the provision of a satisfactory restoration after successful retreatment. Gross caries may determine that a tooth cannot be retreated, and is better extracted (Fig 3-8). If the tooth is not restorable, then it is pointless retreating the tooth.

The restoration must be replaced by an appropriate provisional restoration prior to root canal retreatment if it is:

- deficient
- undergoing significant marginal breakdown
- associated with secondary or recurrent caries.

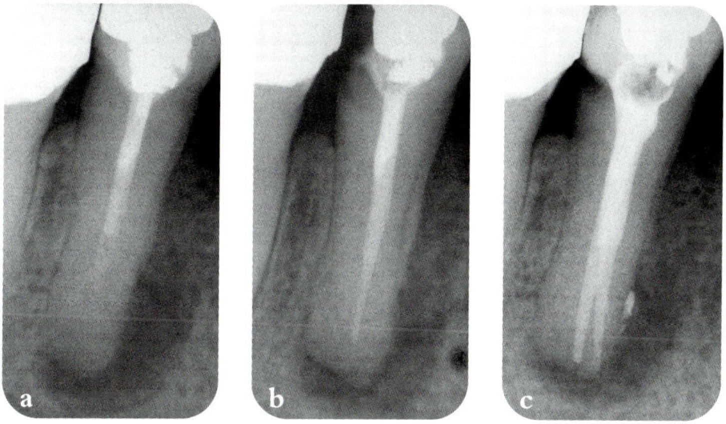

Fig 3-6 Failure according to ESE guidelines. (a) Original root filling. (b) Four years later, the periapical lesion diminished in size but not completely resolved. (c) Following non-surgical retreatment, there are actually two canals.

Fig 3-7 It is vital to ascertain the restorability of a tooth before embarking on retreatment. (a) Pre-op radiograph. (b) Before and (c) after removal of gross caries.

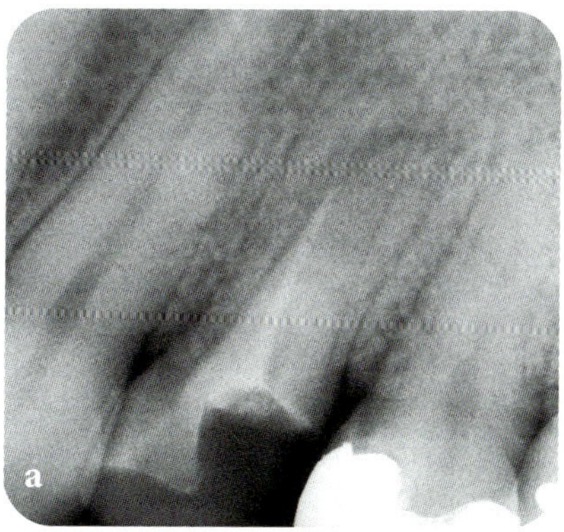

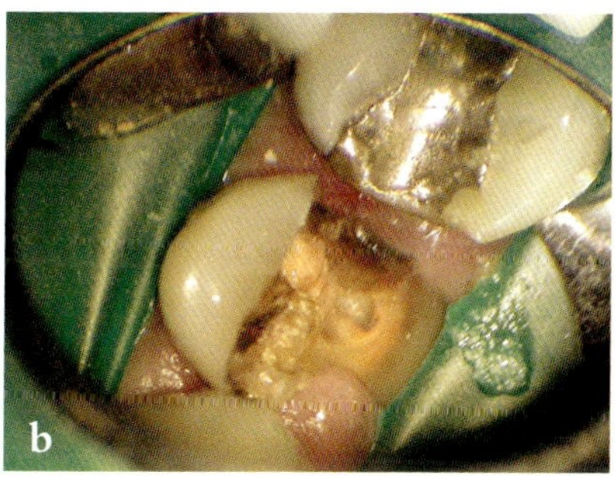

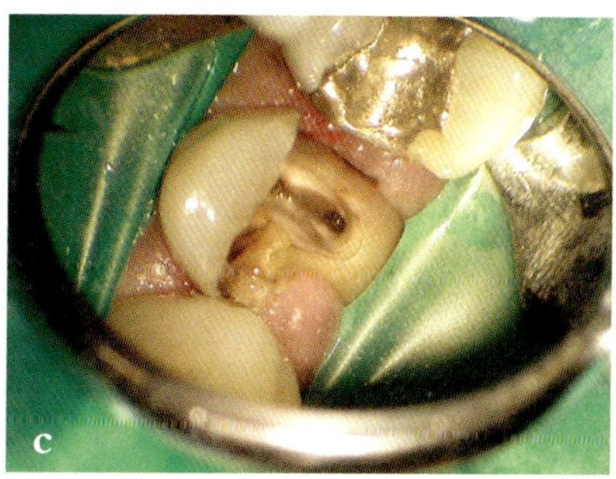

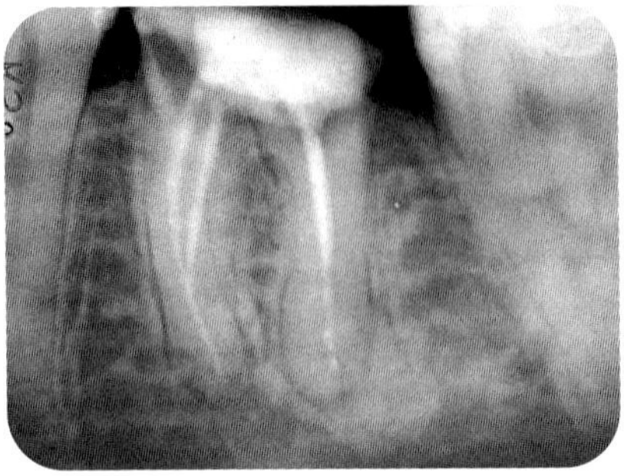

Fig 3-8 Caries may mean a tooth is not restorable and retreatment is pointless.

Regardless of whether a new coronal restoration is placed, it is imperative that while retreatment is in progress success is not compromised by the lack of an adequate coronal seal.

Periodontal Health

Assessment of the periodontal condition of the tooth should include:

- plaque levels
- gingival recession
- tooth mobility
- periodontal probing depths
- any bleeding or suppuration on probing
- crown-to-root ratios
- furcation involvement (Fig 3-9)
- nature of probing defects.

As a sinus tract opening at the gingival margin may mimic periodontal pocketing, it is important to distinguish between the two (Fig 3-10). A sinus tract can be probed at its point of opening and is narrow, whilst periodontal pocketing has a wide opening and can be probed at more than one point along the gingival margin (Fig 3-11).

If an endodontic-periodontal problem (Fig 3-12) is suspected, this may require combined treatment. Periodontal follow-up is always important wherever periodontal disease activity is evident. Sometimes, it is essential to seek a specialist periodontal opinion if the periodontal support is severely compromised and retreatment although feasible may not help prolong the service life of a tooth. Needless to say, if there is advanced periodontal disease and the tooth has a poor prognosis, it may be better extracted (Fig 3-13).

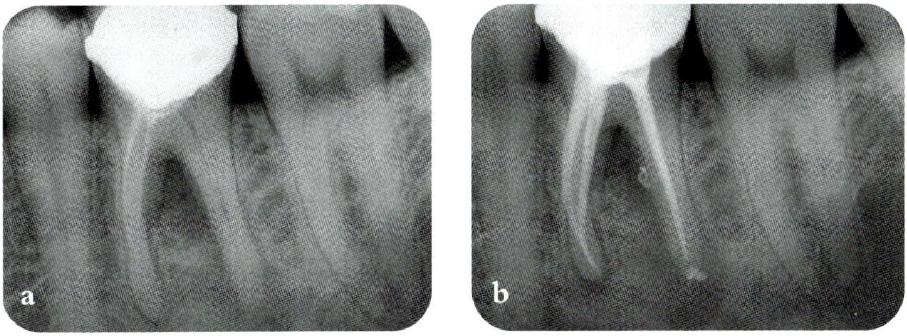

Fig 3-9 Endodontic failure leading to furcation involvement. (a) Pre-op radiograph. (b) Post-op radiograph.

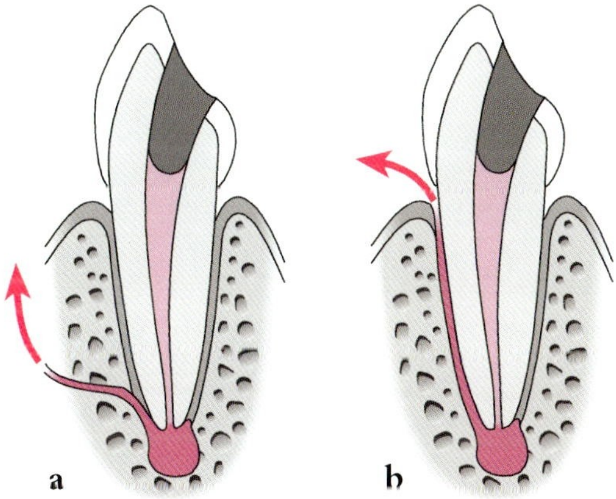

Fig 3-10 A sinus tract may be due to infection tracking: (a) through bone and mucosa or (b) via the periodontal ligament space, opening at the gingival margin.

Fig 3-11 Periodontal probing to help distinguish between a sinus tract opening at the gingival margin as opposed to periodontal pocketing.

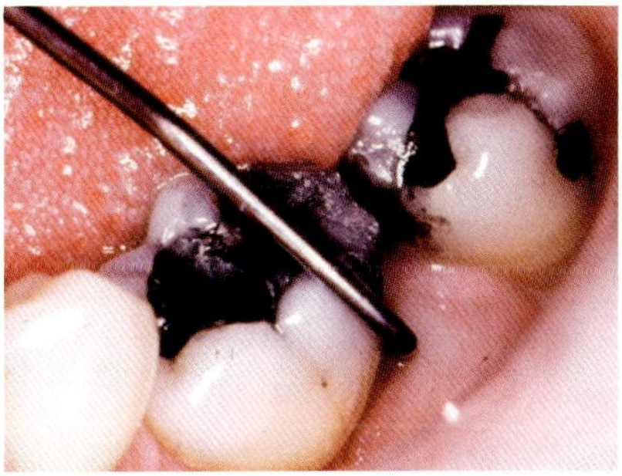

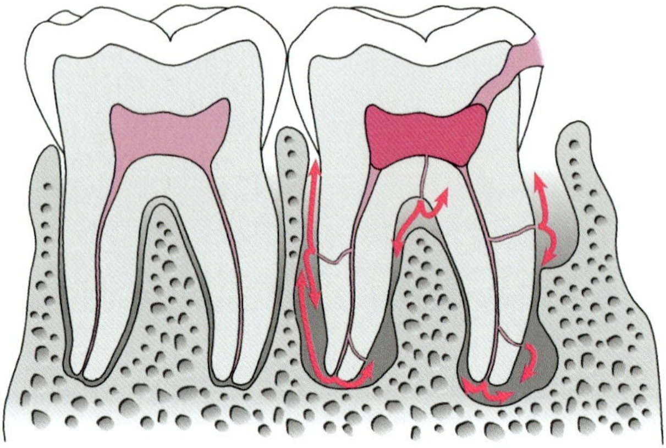

Fig 3-12 Endodontic-periodontal problem.

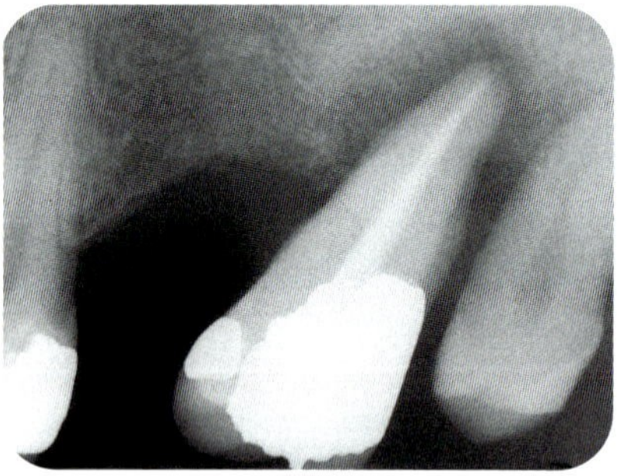

Fig 3-13 Hopeless prognosis because of advanced periodontal disease.

Equipment

Retreatment is more complicated than initial root canal treatment as it involves having to achieve coronal access, removal of the previous root filling and correction of any technical difficulties encountered. Teeth with complex coronal restorations, curved canals (Fig 3-14), canals with ledges and blockages are particularly difficult to retreat. Special equipment may be needed to accomplish the retreatment of such cases. It is unwise to attempt retreatment if the necessary equipment or expertise is not available.

It is claimed that "what you can see, you can do". Unfortunately, "what you can't see or do, makes you frustrated", and magnification with enhanced illumination is especially helpful in retreatment. Magnifying binocular loupes (e.g. SurgiTel, General Scientific Corp., Ann Arbor, MI, USA) can help enhance

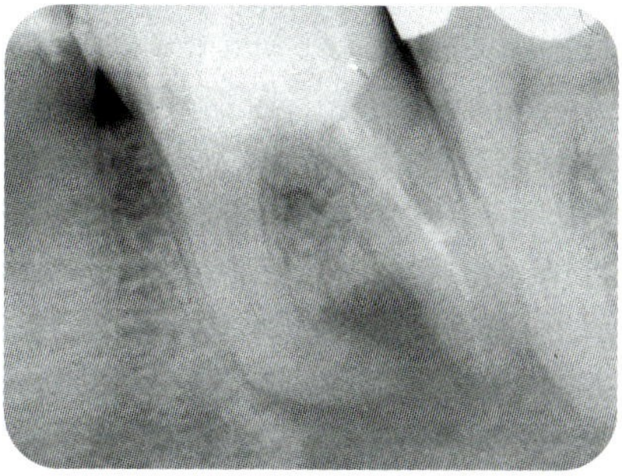

Fig 3-14 Non-surgical retreatment of curved canals is a real challenge.

vision while fibreoptic lighting provides better illumination (Fig 3-15). Dedicated dental operating microscopes (e.g. Global Microscope, Global Surgical Corp., St. Louis, MO, USA) (Fig 3-16) have the combined benefits of magnification and illumination. In surgical retreatment (Chapter 8) magnification has lead to the introduction of microsurgical concepts and techniques. Although an operating microscope may currently be an unrealistic acquisition for most general practices, magnification even with the simplest pair of loupes offers real advantages, and not just in endodontic procedures.

Ultrasound is employed in many retreatment situations. There are two main types of ultrasonic devices on the market: piezo-electric (e.g. Piezon-Mas

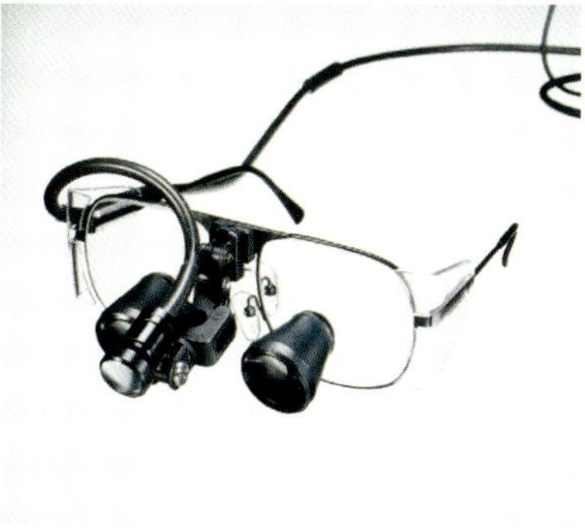

Fig 3-15 Magnifying binocular loupes and fibreoptic light enhances vision and provides better illumination.

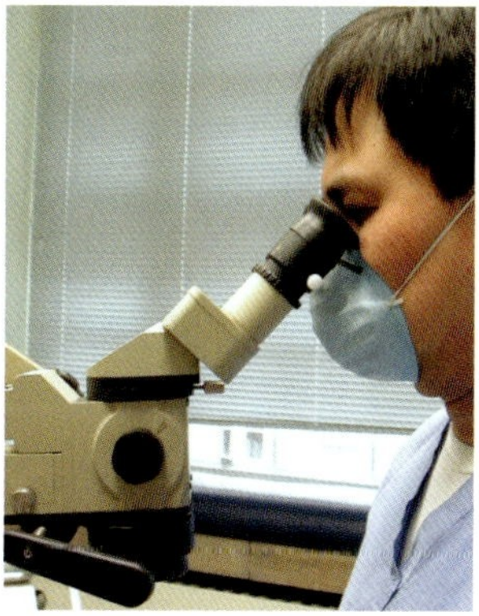

Fig 3-16 Dedicated dental operating microscope.

ter 400, EMS, Le Sentier, Switzerland) (Fig 3-17a) and magnetostrictive (e.g. Cavi-Endo, Dentsply, Weybridge, Surrey, UK) (Fig 3-17b), denoting the way in which the ultrasound is generated. Generally, the piezo-electric systems are better investments, producing more power and allowing wet and dry work in a range of situations. Powerful ultrasound has been one of the key developments in the endodontic retreatment armamentarium.

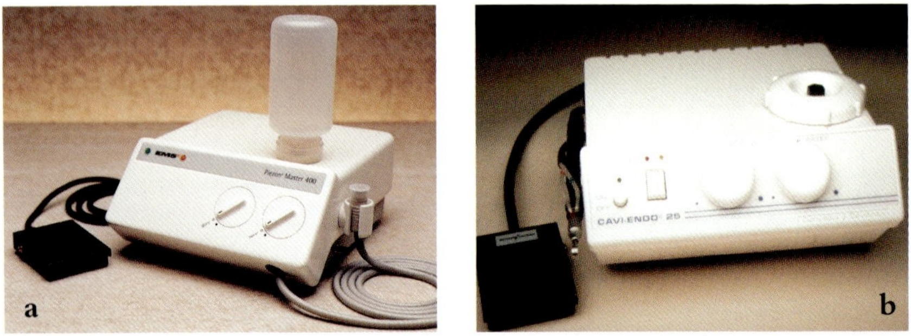

Fig 3-17 Ultrasonic devices. (a) Piezo-electric. (b) Magnetostrictive.

Experience

Some endodontic retreatment procedures are relatively simple, but cases of increasing complexity (Table 3-1) bring challenges which may be best tackled by those with experience of advanced techniques (Fig 3-18). Complex endodontic surgery, should not, for example, be considered a procedure appropriate for inexperienced operators.

When problems are anticipated, referral to a specialist, if possible, may be an option; such cases include:

- uncertain diagnosis
- extremely limited access
- multiple technical problems
- therapy-resistant lesions
- previous unsuccessful retreatment
- complicated surgery
- complex medical history
- anxious patients.

Where specialist services are not available, options may include continuing observation, an attempt to do the best possible for a fully informed and consenting patient or, in some cases, extraction.

Table 3-1 **Non-surgical retreatment: degree of difficulty depending on case scenario**

	Relatively Easy	Moderately Difficult	Extremely Difficult
Crown	Remove and new replacement	Retreat through and repair	Remove intact and reuse
Posts	Non-metallic Possible to drill out	Metallic Tapered Smooth-sided Conventional cement Regular size	Metallic Parallel-sided Threaded Adhesive cement Oversized
RFM			
Gutta percha	Loose, single cone, or poorly condensed	Well-condensed	Overextended
Silver point	Good access Coronal extension	Good access No coronal extension	Restricted access No coronal extension
Cement or paste	Non-setting, soft	Semi-solid, soluble	Hard and dense, not soluble

* RFM, root filling material

Patient's Expectations and Cooperation

The patient's expectations and cooperation must be taken into account. Attitudes to periapical disease vary and a patient's subjective and personal values may influence their preference or otherwise for intervention. A patient who does not wish to have a root canal retreatment or does not appreciate the need, may prefer a hands-off approach. Nevertheless, the patient should always be given a full explanation and time to consider the disease and its risks, what retreatment entails and the possible sequelae, the likely cost and alternative treatment options. Medicolegally, the patient has to give consent and if the patient refuses this, it has to be respected and noted in the patient's records. The patient's and dentist's expectations should match each other's to make retreatment a worthwhile exercise.

patient's expectations + cooperation = dentist's expectations + capabilities

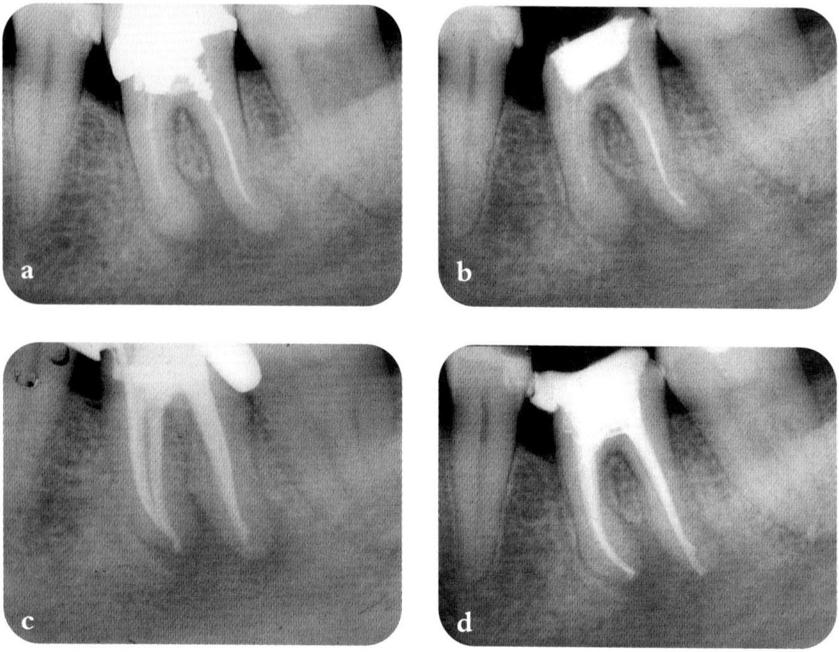

Fig 3-18 Complicated cases demand experience in advanced techniques. (a) Before and (b) after an attempt at non-surgical retreatment; (c) subsequent to specialist referral and (d) completed retreatment.

Cost

In an ideal world, cost would have no influence on treatment planning. In reality, however, cost may be a prime consideration. Practitioners may therefore be faced with the extremely difficult ethical dilemma of having to decide whether to attempt retreatment if the cost involved is greater than the remuneration available; such tensions are an unfortunate reality in everyday clinical practice.

Costs may be considered as (Fig 3-19):

- Direct - retreatment fee, cost of any medication and new restoration.
- Indirect - loss of income, often for lengthy treatment and travel costs to a secondary referral centre.
- Intangible - any pain and suffering involved.

Every effort should be made to prevent the loss of any functional tooth that is of immediate and future value to the patient. As part of the decision-making

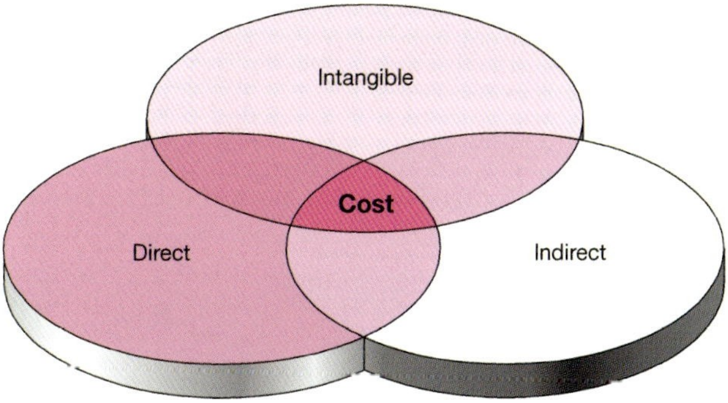

Fig 3-19 The cost of retreatment.

process, the cost/benefit should be weighed against alternative options (Fig 3-20). Whilst an extraction may be a more expedient and less costly option than retreatment in the short term, the subsequent prosthetic replacement may involve more lengthy and costly interventions and long-term restorative options may also be compromised by future direct and intangible costs.

cost of retreatment + restoration ≤ cost of extraction + replacement

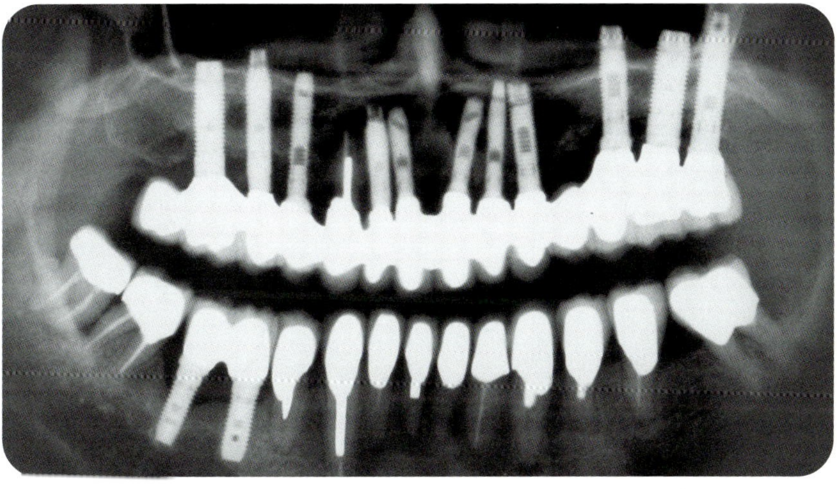

Fig 3-20 Endodontics or implants? The cost/benefit should be considered carefully.

Risk of Complications and Probability of Biological Healing
The risk of complications associated with retreatment both local and systemic must be assessed.

Systemic
As part of risk analysis, preoperative assessment must include the patient's medical history, together with details of any medication. Retreatment is not contraindicated in patients with a history or risk of endocarditis provided the biological objectives (see Chapter 4) can be satisfactorily completed and there is realistic expectation of eliminating infection and achieving healing. Every case should, however, be considered individually, in consultation where necessary with the patient's medical practitioner and relevant medical specialists.

Local
Instrument breakage, perforation and other procedural accidents may occur when trying to remove the previous root filling. Tissue scarring and nerve injury may occur as a result of surgical retreatment. Just as a patient should be informed about what can be done to save a tooth with a failed root canal treatment, the patient should also be advised of possible complications of retreatment. If the potential risks outweigh the benefits, then retreatment is probably not advisable (Fig 3-21). Many factors considered earlier will impact on such decisions. Apart from the equipment, skill and experience of the operator, different dentists will have varying perceptions on the probability of success in individual cases. It must be emphasized that the consequences of not retreating a tooth must be considered against the probability of securing healing.

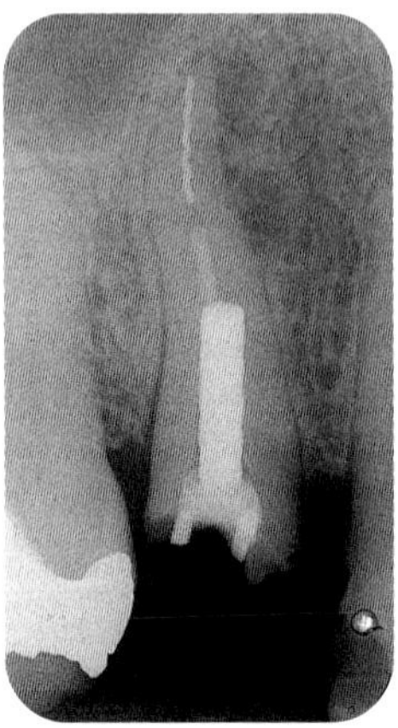

Fig 3-21 If the potential risk of complications is high and probability of biological healing low, then retreatment is not advisable.

Non-Surgical Versus Surgical Retreatment

Once it is agreed that a tooth should be retreated, it must be decided whether to approach the problem non-surgically or surgically. It is axiomatic that:

"When failure has occurred after root canal treatment, surgical retreatment should not be chosen as the first treatment option until the possibility of non-surgical retreatment has been ruled out."

How Do We Choose the Right Approach?

Compared with non-surgical retreatment, surgical retreatment:

- may be more expedient
- radiological healing may be evident earlier

but:

- surgery is a more radical procedure
- the outcome is less predictable
- risk of late failure is higher.

It is clear from the literature that the long-term success of surgical retreatment is no better than that of well-executed non-surgical retreatment. Additionally, the early tissue response after commencing non-surgical retreatment provides a good indication of the likelihood of success. For example, a sinus tract which has been present for months or years will often disappear within days of cleaning and disinfecting the root canal system (Fig 3-22).

Therefore, if a tooth has a simple restoration, is crowned, or is a bridge abutment, an initial attempt should be made to retreat the tooth conventionally. Only if this proves unsuccessful or if the results are unsatisfactory should a surgical approach be considered. Expedient oral surgical referral was once considered an acceptable approach for any failing case, but current understanding of the disease and the limitations of surgery have changed this view. Although oral surgery referrals remain an option, do not be surprised if a case is returned for non-surgical retreatment.

Even posts, in a majority of cases, are no barrier to the non-surgical approach. If a post crown is present, wherever feasible, the post should be removed and non-surgical retreatment instituted. To carry out surgery in the hope of incarcerating the microorganisms within the root canal system is futile (Fig 3-23); unless the reservoir of infection is eliminated, it may continue to cause periapical inflammation adjacent to the resected root face. In addition, non-surgical retreatment after post removal is more con-

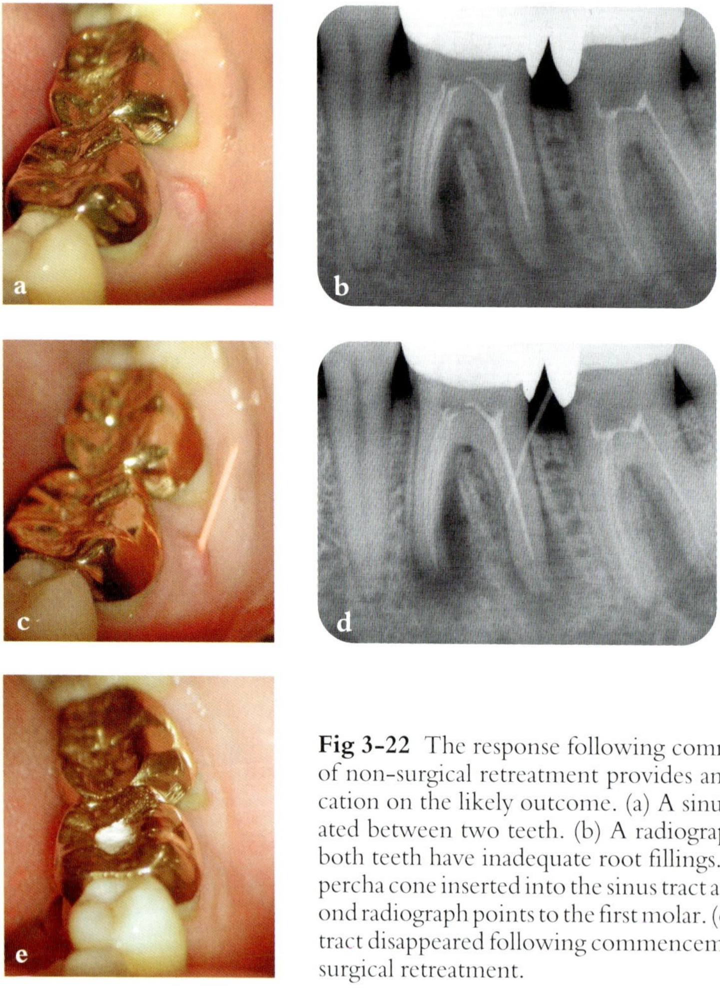

Fig 3-22 The response following commencement of non-surgical retreatment provides an early indication on the likely outcome. (a) A sinus tract situated between two teeth. (b) A radiograph showing both teeth have inadequate root fillings. (c) A gutta percha cone inserted into the sinus tract and (d) a second radiograph points to the first molar. (e) The sinus tract disappeared following commencement of non-surgical retreatment.

servative and does not reduce root length and compromise the crown:root ratio (see Chapter 8).

If a recalcitrant infection is suspected, the initial approach is still to retreat the tooth. If, despite a technically pleasing retreatment result, the tooth still has signs and symptoms of disease, then the problem may be due to a refractory lesion. Surgical retreatment may be needed but there is also the possibility that the tooth may not be salvageable.

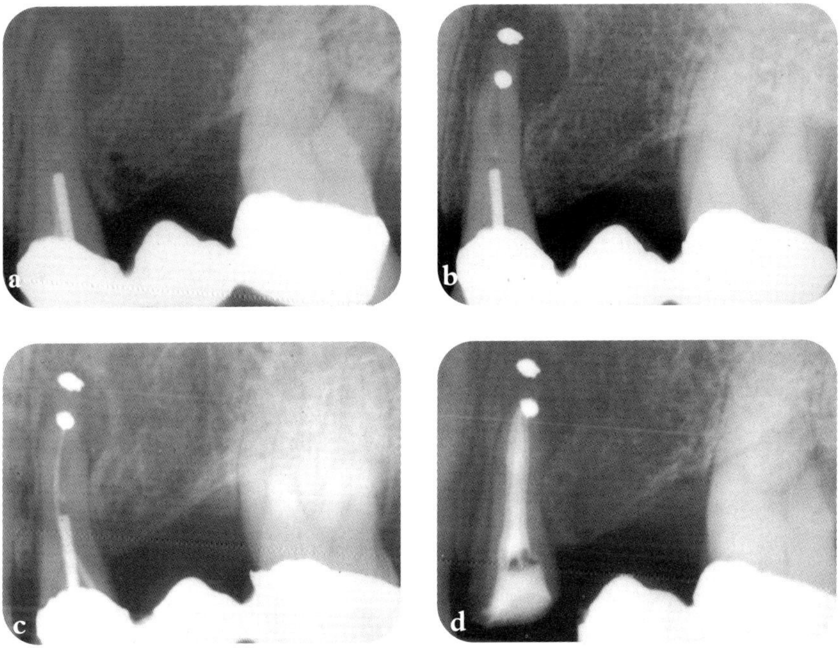

Fig 3-23 Surgery in the hope of incarcerating the microorganisms within the root canal system is futile. (a) A bridge supporting premolar tooth needing treatment. (b) Since a post was present, an apicectomy and root-end filling was carried out. (c) Failure about a year later; radiograph with a gutta percha cone in the sinus tract. (d) The bridge was sectioned, crown and post removed, and non-surgical retreatment performed.

Where the previous root canal filling cannot be removed by any available means, or a non-surgical approach carries an unacceptable risk of causing irreversible damage to the tooth for example, risk of root fracture removing a large post - then a surgical approach may be preferable (Fig 3-24). In a few cases - the tooth may be better extracted, while others may require a combination of non-surgical followed by surgical retreatment.

Success is dependent on careful case selection and deciding on the correct retreatment approach; the indications for retreatment will be considered next.

When to Treat?

Technical Deficiency

If failure has occurred simply because canals were inadequately cleaned, shaped, filled or protected coronally as evidenced from the quality and quan-

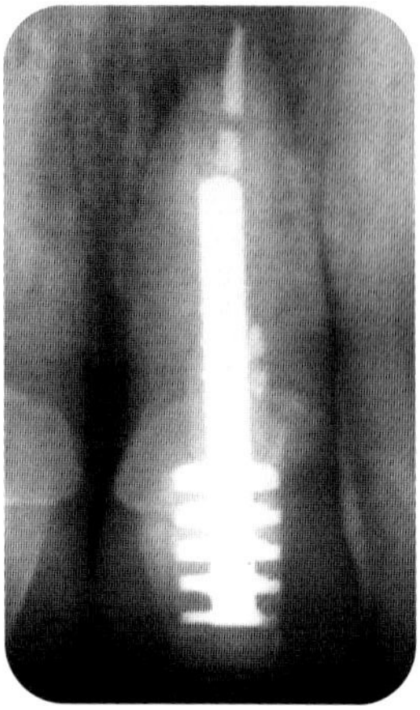

Fig 3-24 Surgery is indicated if non-surgical retreatment is not feasible or risky.

tity of the existing root canal filling, then non-surgical retreatment is indicated (Fig 3-25). The result will normally be successful and there is seldom a need to resort to surgery.

If failure has occurred because of a missed canal, non-surgical retreatment is indicated to locate and treat the untreated canal. In multirooted teeth, it is prudent to retreat all the canals, not just the missed or inadequately treated canals.

This approach ensures that the entire root canal system and any communicating channels are thoroughly cleaned and that a good-quality root filling is placed under optimal asepsis in every canal. It also eliminates the possibility that origi-

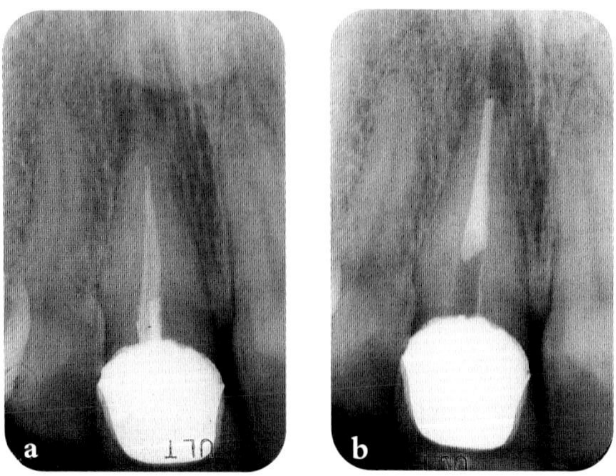

Fig 3-25 Technically deficient root filling: non-surgical retreatment indicated in the first instance. (a) Pre-op radiograph. (b) Post-op radiograph.

nally treated canals may not be as adequate as they appeared during case assessment.

Procedural Errors

Non-surgical root canal retreatment should be considered if during the original root canal treatment any of the following occurred:

- an obstruction
- a ledge
- a perforation
- an instrument fracture.

An attempt should be made to:

- remove or bypass the obstruction (Fig 3-26)
- close off the perforation
- negotiate the root canal to its full working length and treat the entire root canal system.

If this proves impossible or if the non-surgical retreatment result is deemed to be less than satisfactory, then remedial surgery may be needed at a later date. In rare instances, it may be better to extract the tooth rather than attempt surgery if the damage is beyond repair or the prognosis is poor, in particular, when the tooth is intended to be part of a complicated restoration.

Pain, Swelling, Sinus Tract

Pain, swelling or the presence of a draining sinus tract are common features of endodontic failure (Fig 3-27). Often, a small and episodically active sinus

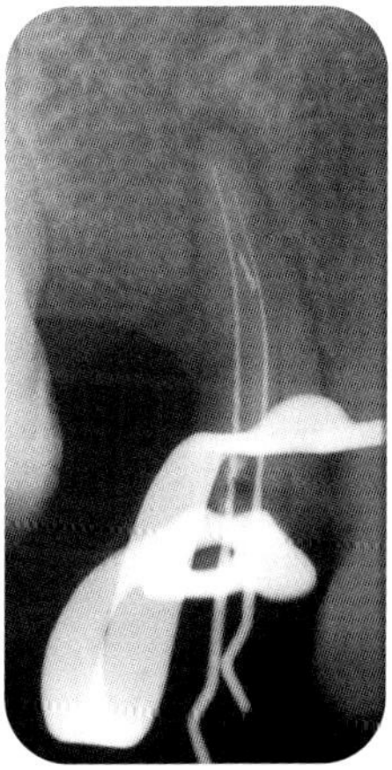

Fig 3-26 Even if a fractured instrument is present, non-surgical retreatment should be attempted, to remove or bypass the retained instrument.

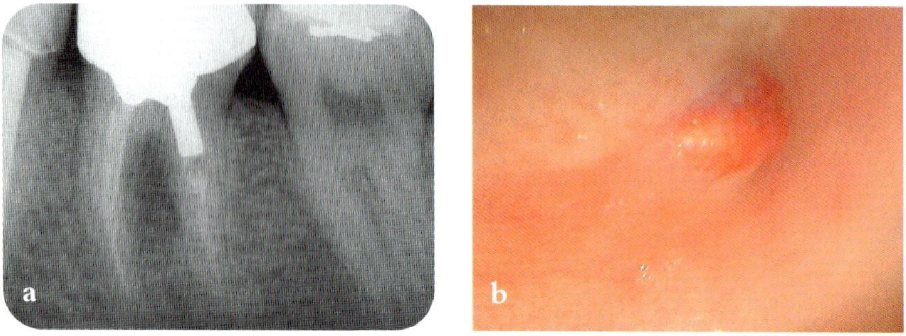

Fig 3-27 Indicators of failure. (a) Radiograph of tooth which was tender to bite. (b) Same tooth with localised swelling.

tract is the only sign of disease and causes the patient little concern, but the presence of active infection should not be ignored, as the condition will not improve with time. It is preferable to institute treatment before acute symptoms develop, rather than leave a smouldering infection, which may jeopardise the long-term survival of the tooth. Perhaps as important are the growing concerns about possible links between chronic dental infections and systemic maladies. By today's standard, from the clinician's viewpoint, it is not acceptable to leave evidently active infection unattended, whether troublesome and symptomatic or not.

Persistent Symptoms

Sometimes, patients may continue to experience symptoms from an apparently well root treated tooth. Needless to say, non-dental causes should first be excluded. If the radiograph of the tooth and its root filling appear adequate and there is no obvious cause for failure, then retreatment should be considered in the first instance. There is usually a logical reason for failure although the cause may not be immediately clear or elude diagnosis (Fig 3-28). Possible reasons include:

- convert coronal microleakage
- undetected cracked tooth
- part of the root canal system untreated
- recalcitrant infection.

Retreatment on this basis can be viewed as a diagnostic procedure, with a favourable early response confirming or refuting the suspected reason for failure. If there is no means of knowing the reason for non-healing or residual symptoms, then the first step is still to retreat the tooth. To do

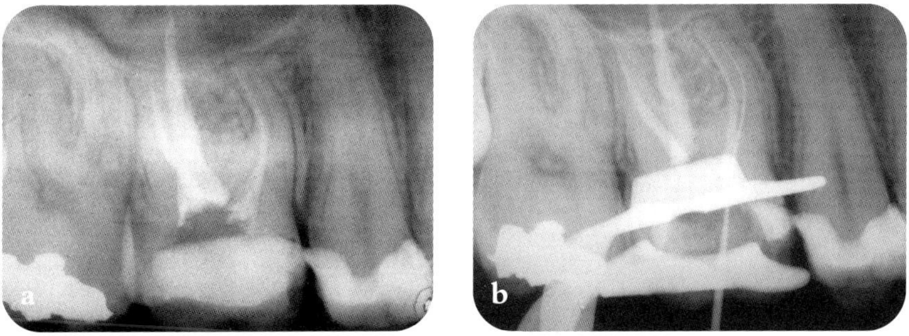

Fig 3-28 The reason for failure may not be immediately obvious. (a) An apparently well-treated maxillary first molar. (b) Unfortunately, there was an untreated, missed second mesiobuccal canal.

nothing in these cases is to expect patients to live with the persistent symptoms. At the other extreme, to extract the tooth without attempting retreatment is to condemn the tooth without giving it a second chance.

New Coronal Restoration

Where the coronal restoration is scheduled for replacement and leakage has exposed the underlying root filling to the mouth, root canal retreatment may be an essential foundation-laying step. Studies have shown that when coronal leakage occurs, even filled canals become contaminated very quickly, especially if the root filling is technically inadequate.

Similarly, even when there is no overt coronal leakage, existing root canal filling should be checked before new crowns or bridges are provided. Teeth with root fillings of questionable quality should be considered carefully for retreatment (Fig 3-29). Although it is tempting to accept a less than adequate root filling, in particular if the tooth is symptom-free, it is prudent to retreat beforehand to avoid the possibility of embarrassing failure, typically soon after the new restoration is placed. The remedial costs in these cases may be great in direct, indirect, intangible and medicolegal terms. A new restoration failing because of a poor root filling is not a practice builder and certainly not what patients expect. In short, it is usually better to retreat a tooth if there are any doubts rather than accept the endodontic inadequacies and risk failure after placement of a new restoration. Again, the costs and benefits of intervention should be carefully weighed.

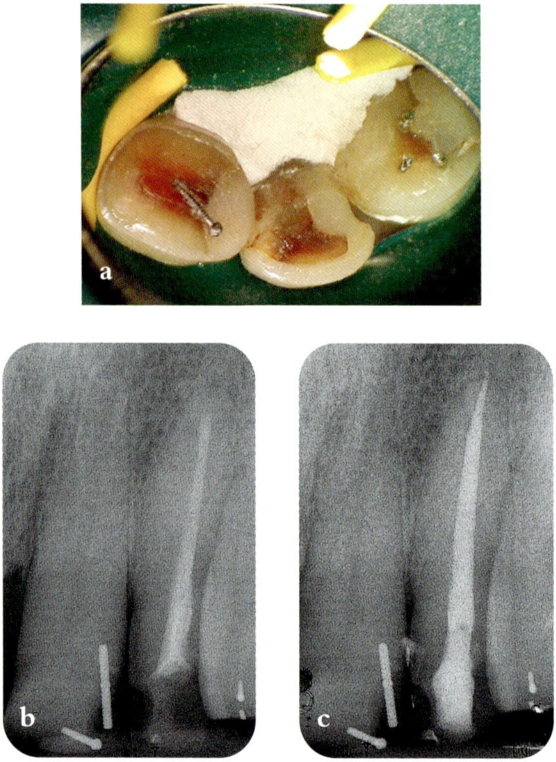

Fig 3-29 If a new restoration is planned, an inadequate root filling should be revised even if the tooth is symptom-free. (a) Crowns planned to replace existing pin-retained composite restorations. (b) The root filling in the lateral incisor could be improved. (c) Following non-surgical retreatment.

When Not to Treat?

Some teeth may have an inadequate root filling and may not be considered a success according to stringent criteria (Fig 3-30). No immediate action is indicated, however, if:

- the patient is symptom-free and not at systemic risk
- there are no obvious signs of active infection
- a new restoration is not planned
- it is not a strategic tooth within a broader plan of care
- retreatment entails an unacceptably high risk of complications
- retreatment is unlikely to be successful.

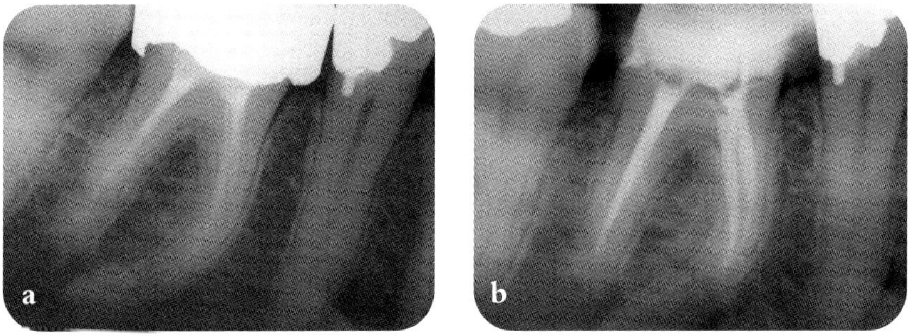

Fig 3-30 Immediate action may not be necessary until a change of circumstances. (a) An inadequate root filling in a heavily restored but symptom-free tooth. (b) Non-surgical retreatment prior to provision of a crown.

If no immediate intervention is contemplated, the tooth should be reviewed periodically and the patient advised to be in contact if they have any concerns. It must be emphasized that this is not an excuse for supervised neglect. Further developments, particularly active symptoms, may dictate the need for action.

Conclusions

- A major part of managing endodontic failures revolves around the decision-making process.
- Clinical decision-making is a complicated process and is influenced by many factors which must be balanced with care.
- The clinician has the difficult task of weighing the risk/benefit, cost/benefit and success/failure ratios as part of rational decision-making.
- Comprehensive examination and careful case selection are important when deciding on intervention; most teeth are amenable to retreatment but some are not.
- Non-surgical rather than surgical retreatment should be considered first when failure has occurred.
- Sometimes, immediate intervention may not be necessary for failed endodontic cases but infection which is obvious to the patient or dentist should never be ignored.

Further Reading

Danin J, Strömberg T, Forsgren H, et al. Clinical management of nonhealing periradicular pathosis. Surgery versus endodontic retreatment. Oral Surg Oral Med Oral Pathol Oral Radiol Endod 1996;82:213-217.

Friedman S. Considerations and concepts of case selection in the management of post-treatment endodontic disease (endodontic failure). Endod Topics 2002;1:54-78.

Hepworth MJ, Friedman S. Treatment outcome of surgical versus non-surgical management of endodontic failures. J Cand Dent Assoc 1997;63:364-371.

Kvist T. Endodontic retreatment. Aspects of decision making and clinical outcome. Swedish Dental J 2001;(Suppl 144).

Molven O, Halse H, Grung B. Surgical management of endodontic failures: indications and treatment results. Int Endod J 1991;41:33-42.

Nehammer CF, Chong BS, Rattan R. Endodontics. Clin Risk 2004;10:45-48.

Chapter 4

Biological Objectives of Retreatment

Aim

To review the biological objectives of retreatment and how they may be attained to transform failure into successful healing.

Outcome

At the end of this chapter, the practitioner should have a clear understanding of what they are trying to achieve when they retreat a failed endodontic case, and be conversant with the treatment measures necessary to gain success.

Introduction

The primary aim of root canal treatment is the elimination and future exclusion of infection from the root canal system (Fig 4-1). Endodontic failures usually result from failure to achieve this primary aim and retreatment is intended to correct the inadequacies of initial treatment.

The Microbial Flora

The microbial flora of infected root canals is complex. Depending on whether it is a primary or secondary infection, it may consist of cocci, rods (Fig 4-2),

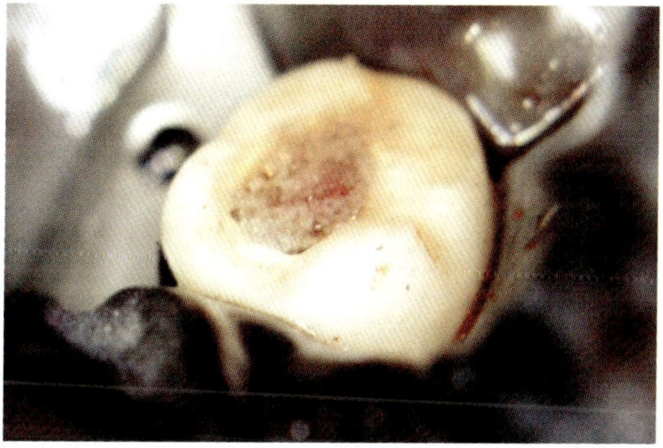

Fig 4-1 The primary aim of root canal treatment is the elimination and future exclusion of infection of the root canal system.

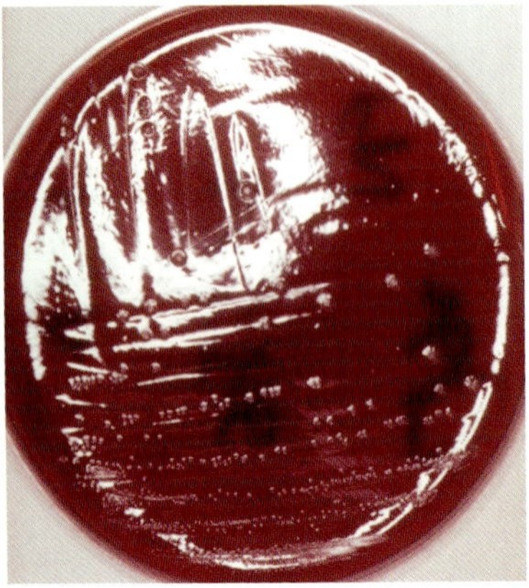

Fig 4-2 Blood agar culture of *Fusobacterium nucleatum*, a rod-shaped endodontic pathogen.

Fig 4-3 Dentinal tubules invaded by bacteria, labelled with special stain.

spirochaetes, filaments and fungi, often maintaining each other in ecological and nutritional relationships. They may exist in two forms:

- planktonic – loose collections or suspensions of microorganisms within the root canal lumen
- biofilm – dense aggregates, forming plaques on and within the root canal dentine wall.

Microbes may also invade the tubular structure of the dentine walls (Fig 4-3) to depths of 300 μm or more.

Elimination of Microorganisms

Elimination of microorganisms from the root canal system is normally accomplished by:

- mechanical instrumentation
- chemical antimicrobial agents, including irrigants and medicaments.

Exclusion of New Microbial Infection

Microorganisms can be prevented from entering the cleaned root canal system by ensuring a "total canal seal" by placing a:

- complete root canal filling (apical seal) and
- coronal restoration (coronal seal).

All elements of the process are important in ensuring success.

apical seal + coronal seal = total canal seal

Fulfilling the Biological Objectives

It is not the intention of this chapter to revise basic endodontic skills; these are covered in the first book of the series, *Rational Root Canal Treatment in Practice*. However, to fulfil the biological objectives of retreatment, a number of practical considerations and recommendations are reinforced.

Aseptic Treatment Regime

Tooth isolation using rubber dam (Fig 4-4) should be considered as mandatory for all endodontic procedures, in accordance with the principles of controlled asepsis. To guard against unplanned fracture, teeth with severe coronal tissue loss, heavy occlusion contacts or with cracks must be relieved from significant occlusal loading and protected, even in the short-term, by placing an orthodontic band (Fig 4-5) or temporary crown. The temporary restoration should additionally prevent recontamination of the root canal system by precluding the ingress of oral fluids and microorganisms.

Access

A tooth cannot be retreated until the canal system is re-entered.

Coronal access

The first obstacle to overcome is to enter the pulp chamber and uncover the root canal filling. This entails getting past the coronal restoration and any underlying core material, including posts.

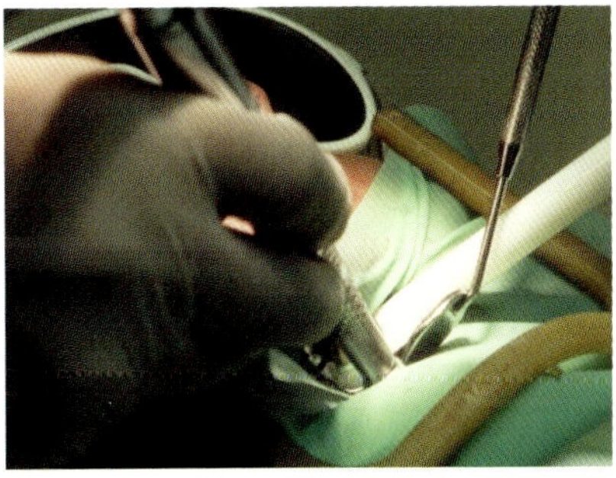

Fig 4-4 Rubber dam is mandatory for all endodontic procedures.

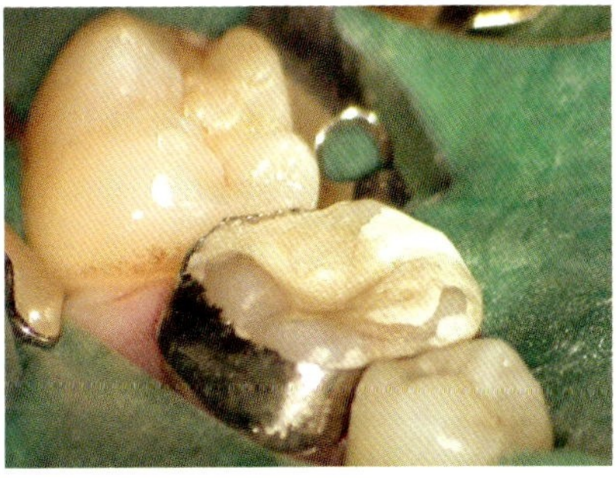

Fig 4-5 Orthodontic band placed to protect a structurally fragile tooth.

Radicular access
The next obstacle is whatever may be obstructing instrumentation of the whole canal system including the root filling material. The task is to clear the root canal system so that it is negotiable to its terminus, to enable recleaning, reshaping and refilling so as to achieve and preserve periapical health. The retreatment techniques to gain coronal and radicular access will be covered in Chapters 5 and 6, respectively.

Mechanical Instrumentation
In primary treatment, the goals of mechanical preparation are to:
- thoroughly clean
- adequately shape the canal system.

In retreatment, previous efforts may have resulted in:
- underpreparation
- overpreparation
- a combination of both, in different parts of the root canal system.

Whether the root canal system is underprepared or overprepared, it should be recleaned and redisinfected, to remove microorganisms and pulpal remnants.

If the canals are underprepared, they should be shaped to produce a smooth, continuously tapered preparation, widest coronally and narrowest at the apical terminus. The shape should allow effective penetration of the root canal irrigant and placement of a good-quality root filling.

If the root canals are overprepared, they should be reshaped so that a retentive form is reestablished to contain the root filling. Heavy planning of fragile canals walls is often unnecessary for effective cleaning; wherever possible, valuable tooth tissue should always be conserved.

Accurate determination of working length is as important in retreatment as in primary treatment to:
- correct the previous deficiencies of cleaning and shaping
- avoid injuring the periapical tissues
- prevent further, or correct existing, procedural errors
- confine the root filling within the root canal system.

The apical limit for root canal procedures is generally accepted to be the apical constriction. In cases where there is chronic infection, inflammatory api-

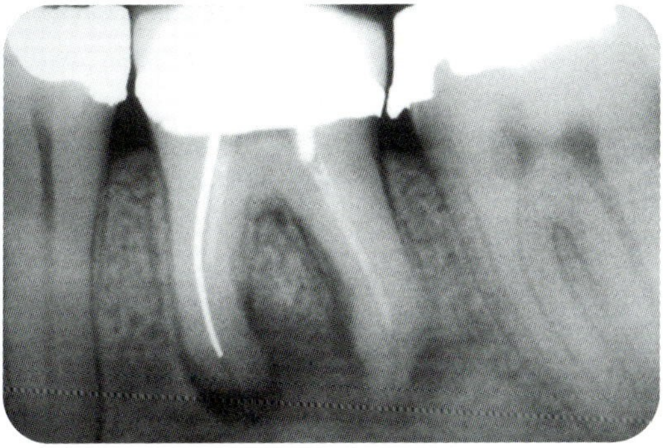

Fig 4-6 Inflammatory apical root resorption due to chronic infection may destroy the natural contours of the periapex.

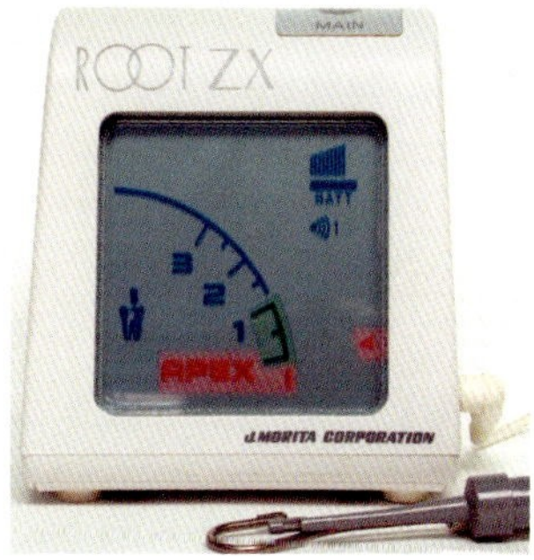

Fig 4-7 Dual frequency apex locator.

cal root resorption (Fig 4-6) may have destroyed the natural contours of the periapex, making it difficult to determine accurately the canal length. An electronic apex locator is helpful in these cases, but the canal length should be verified by taking the necessary radiographs. New generations of gradient impedance apex locators (e.g. Root ZX, Morita, Kyoto, Japan) (Fig 4-7) which employ two or more frequencies are more reliable and less susceptible to inaccuracies caused by the presence of electrolytes (e.g. blood, exudate or irrigant) in the root canal.

Antimicrobial Therapy

Mechanical instrumentation is combined with chemical antimicrobial therapy to eliminate microorganisms from the root canal system.

Root canal irrigant

Irrigants have many roles including:

- washing out canal debris
- dissolving pulpal remnants
- lubricating the canal
- disinfecting the root canal system.

A root canal irrigant may be introduced with an endodontic syringe and needle or an ultrasonic device. If a needle and syringe are used, the endodontic needle, which is blunt-ended with an open side, should not be jammed in, but loosely positioned in the canal. The irrigant is delivered slowly, taking care not to force it beyond the apex. As an additional safety precaution against inadvertent extrusion of irrigant, the index finger (Fig 4-8a) rather than the thumb (Fig 4-8b) should be used to push the plunger of the syringe so that the irrigant is ejected with less hydraulic pressure. Ultrasonic devices for irrigating root canals (see Fig 3-17) are very efficient as large volumes of irrigant can be dispensed with ease and agitated to flush out the canal system thoroughly. Piezo-electric and magnetostrictive ultrasonic units are equally suitable for this purpose.

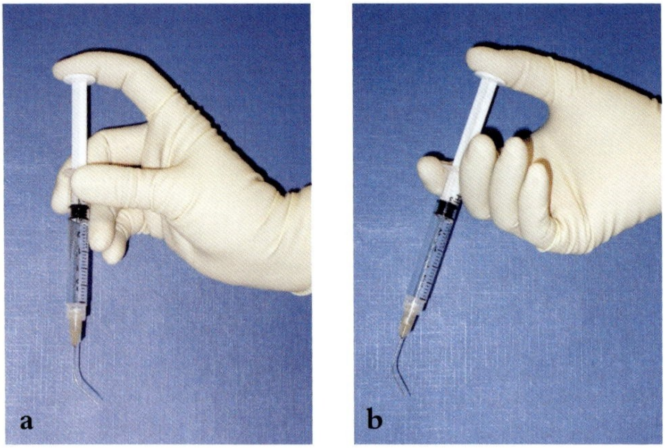

Fig 4-8 Avoiding accidental extrusion of irrigant. (a) The index finger rather than (b) the thumb should be used to push the plunger of the irrigating syringe.

Sodium hypochlorite is considered the most effective endodontic irrigant because of its antimicrobial and tissue solvent properties.

Sodium hypochlorite has a long record of effective and safe use in medicine. As early as 1915, sodium hypochlorite was recommended for irrigation of open, infected wounds. Commercially available sodium hypochlorite solutions, like thin household bleach (Fig 4-9a), typically have a concentration of 4.5% +/- 0.4%. They are very alkaline and hypertonic, and as a root canal irrigant are usually diluted before use. Milton sterilising fluid (Procter & Gamble, Weybridge, Surrey) (Fig 4-9b), a stabilised 1% sodium hypochlorite solution, also contains 16.5% sodium chloride and may be used undiluted as a root canal irrigant.

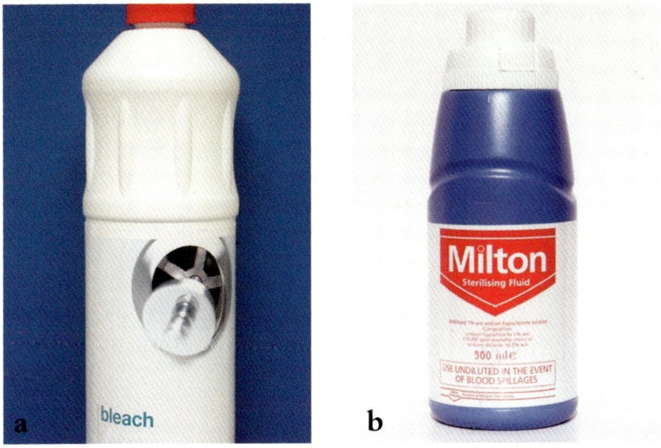

Fig 4-9 Sodium hypochlorite solutions. (a) Household bleach, usually used diluted. (b) Milton sterilising fluid may be used undiluted.

The activity of sodium hypochlorite will deteriorate on storage and as a function of:

- time
- temperature
- exposure to light
- contamination with metallic ions.

There is no agreement on the optimal concentration of sodium hypochlo rite. Concentrations ranging from 0.5–5.25% have been advocated. What is more important is that it is used and in copious amounts.

Chelating agents

A smear layer is produced during canal instrumentation. This amorphous, irregular, tenacious layer consists of organic and inorganic components, together with fragments of odontoblastic processes, microorganisms and pulp tissue. The superficial smear layer is 1–2 μm thick. In the deeper layer, smear plugs are packed into dentinal tubules to depths of up to 40 μm. The smear layer may act as a reservoir for microorganisms and their products. Since the smear layer occludes the orifices of dentinal tubules, it prevents the penetration of irrigants and medicaments into the tubules; it also impedes intimate adaptation and tubular penetration of root filling materials. As these may be considered detrimental, there is an argument for removal. Chelating agents may be used to remove infected smear layer and open dentinal tubules to allow more effective disinfection of the root canal system. Sometimes, failing cases with overprepared canals may require little more than smear layer removal and thorough disinfection to promote healing.

The main ingredient of chelating agents is ethylenediaminetetraacetic acid (EDTA). Chelating agents are available in gel form (Fig 4-10) or as an aqueous solution (Fig 4-11); the former typically also contains either urea peroxide (RC-Prep, Premier Dental Products, King of Prussia, PA, USA) or carbamide peroxide (File-Eze, Ultradent Products Inc., South Jordan, UT, USA; Glyde, Dentsply Maillefer, Ballaigues, Switzerland) and propylene glycol. Some formulations of the aqueous solution may be buffered to a neutral pH (Pulpdent 17% EDTA solution, Pulpdent Corp., Watertown, MA, USA) (Fig 4-11b). Another formulation, EDTAC, contains a quaternary ammonium compound, Cetrimide (cetyltrimethylammonium bromide), an antiseptic and cationic detergent to help reduce surface tension for better canal wetting. The combination of sodium hypochlorite and EDTA also generates effervescence and the release of oxygen (Fig 4-12), which may help to loosen canal debris and destroy anaerobic microorganisms.

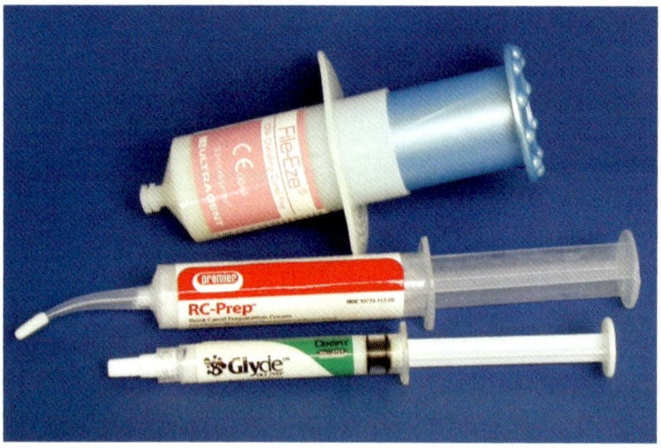

Fig 4-10 Selection of gel-form EDTA products.

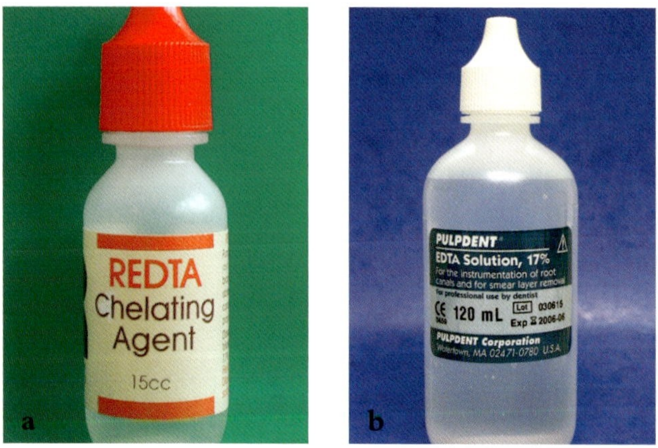

Fig 4-11 Aqueous EDTA solutions. (a) REDTA. (b) Pulpdent.

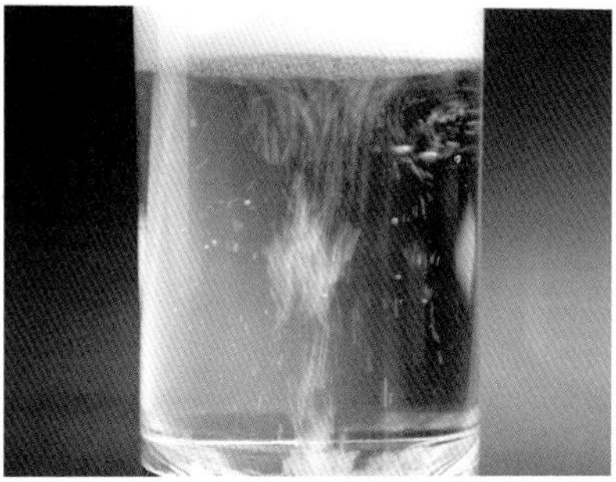

Fig 4-12 The combination of sodium hypochlorite and EDTA generates effervescence and the release of oxygen.

Chelating agents have:
- direct antimicrobial activity
- indirect antimicrobial activity – by opening dentinal tubules to allow better access for irrigants.

Other actions of chelating agents include:
- lubrication
- tissue emulsification
- dentine softening
- keeping debris in suspension.

Other chemicals advocated for smear layer removal, such as simple organic acids, capable of dissolving calcified smear debris but not as easy to use as viscous gel-type EDTA formulations, include:
- citric acid (25%)
- tannic acid (50%)
- polyacrylic acid (40%).

Intracanal medicaments

The role of an intracanal medicament in retreatment is as an antimicrobial agent to eliminate residual microorganisms or at least limit their regrowth. Medicaments are not a substitute for thorough cleaning and adequate shaping of the root canal system, but serve a secondary function.

Calcium hydroxide is a popular intracanal medicament because it:
- has a good spectrum of antimicrobial activity
- has a comparatively long duration of action
- is relatively safe
- is easy to use
- may assist in tissue dissolution.

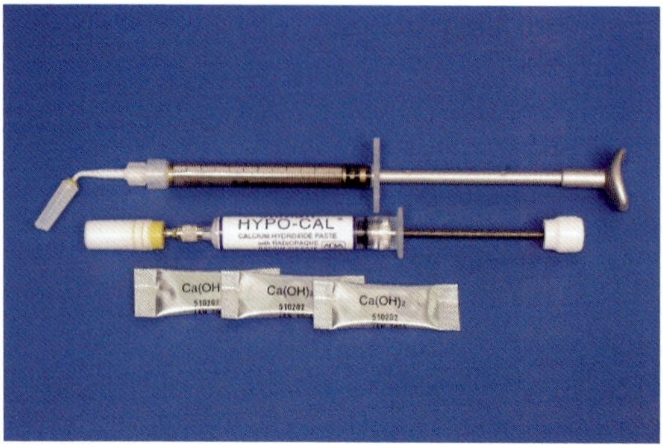

Fig 4-13 Commercially available calcium hydroxide preparations.

Calcium hydroxide is available in ready-to-use commercial preparations (Fig 4-13) or by mixing calcium hydroxide powder with sterile saline, water or local anaesthetic solution. However, it is now recognised that the endodontic flora associated with failed root canal treatments is often quite different from that of untreated teeth. In particular, enteric bacteria are common in retreatment cases, with *Enteroccoccus faecalis* being the most frequent isolate. Yeasts, for example *Candida albicans*, have also been reported to be frequent isolates in failed cases. Unfortunately, calcium hydroxide is less effective in eliminating *E. faecalis*, which is able to withstand the high pH of calcium hydroxide and can survive in environments with minimal available nutrients. The mechanism of its resistance is yet to be clarified, but it is thought it may be due to its ability to invade dentinal tubules and adhere to collagen in the presence of human serum. A functioning proton pump has been reported to be critical to its ability to tolerate a high alkalinity. It has also been reported that *Candida* spp. are resistant to calcium hydroxide. Ideally, a root canal sample should be obtained during retreatment to ascertain the flora, but this is not practicable in everyday clinical practice and the necessary specialist oral microbiological services are rarely available.

For proper antimicrobial management, a multivisit treatment approach involving a period of intracanal dressing may be necessary. If a case fails to respond to thorough cleaning, shaping and, in the first instance, calcium hydroxide medication, a different medicament should be considered. Alternative medicaments advocated for managing such cases and those suspected of being dominated by enterococci include:

- iodine-based compounds, including iodoform-calcium hydroxide combinations (Fig 4-14)
- chlorhexidine
- antibiotic-calcium hydroxide combinations.

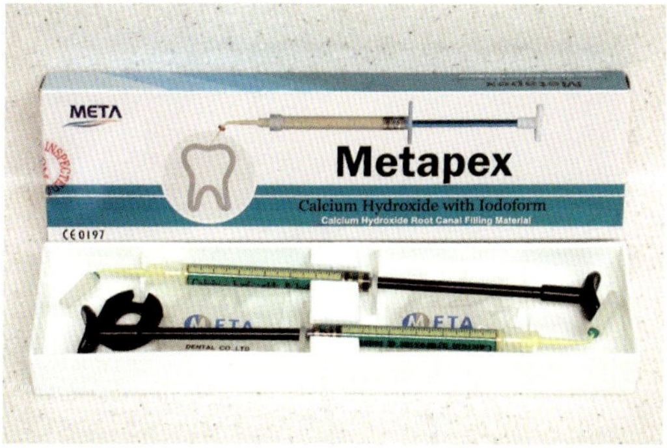

Fig 4-14 Iodoform-calcium hydroxide combination, an alternative intracanal medicament.

There is continuing work to investigate alternative medicaments for recalcitrant cases.

Obturation

Inadequate obturation is a recognised cause of failure, so after thorough cleaning, adequate shaping and effective medication, the root canal system should be completely filled. The root filling should seal all portals of microbial entry.

A gutta percha core combined with a sealer cement is generally considered the most acceptable root filling material. There are, however, countless commercial brands and filling techniques. To ensure a well-performed root filling:

- customise the fit of the master cone – for example, using a gauge or solvent-dip technique (Fig 4-15)
- take a master cone fit radiograph to ascertain its extension and adaptation
- apply heat to soften the material and obtain a more homogenous root filling (Fig 4-16)
- take a radiograph afterwards to check the quality of the root filling and, if necessary, revise the filling.

Sometimes, in wide canals or in cases in which apical damage has occurred, it may be impossible to create an adequate apical retentive form to prevent overfilling. In these cases, Mineral Trioxide Aggregate (MTA) (see Chapter 8), for example, may be used instead of gutta percha as the root filling material (Fig 4-17).

Coronal Temporisation and Restoration

It must not be forgotten that even well-placed root fillings are vulnerable to

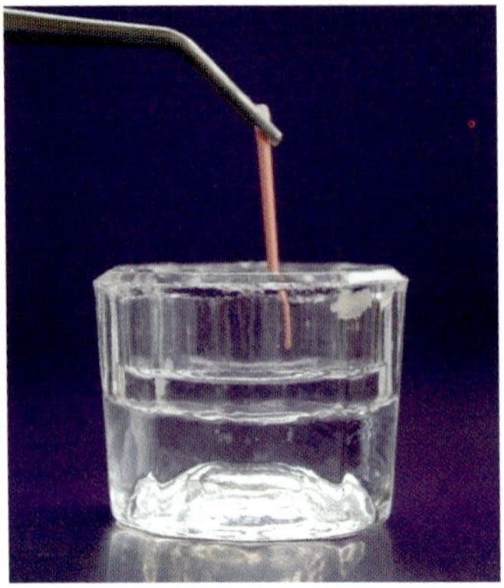

Fig 4-15 Master gutta percha cone customised using the solvent-dip technique.

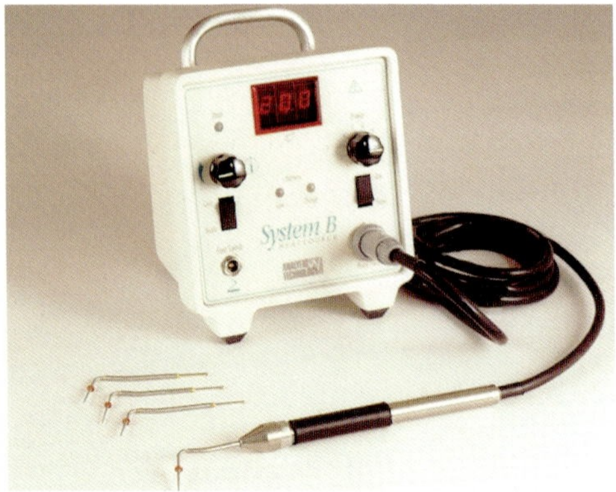

Fig 4-16 Electrically-heated spreaders such as a System B may be used to achieve a more homogenous root filling.

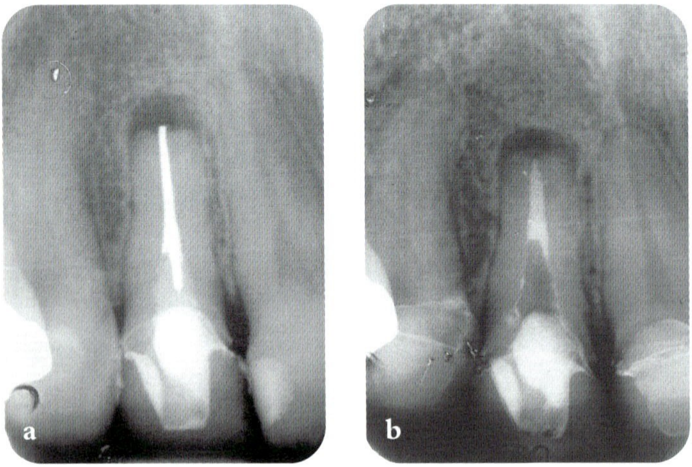

Fig 4-17 Non-surgical retreatment of a silver point root filling. (a) A wide, opened apex due to a previous apicectomy. (b) MTA instead of gutta percha used as root filling. (Courtesy of C. F. Nehammer.)

coronal leakage if the coronal restoration is inadequate. This applies equally to permanent and interim restorations, so care should be taken to prevent coronal leakage. Zinc oxide-eugenol cements have a proven record of preventing microbial leakage, and as a temporary filling will provide the required coronal seal. A reinforced zinc oxide-eugenol cement (IRM or Kalzinol,

Dentsply DeTrey-DeDent, Konstanz, Germany) is superior because it is less likely to disintegrate under functional loading.

The correlation between the prevalence of apical periodontitis and the quality of the root filling and restoration has been investigated by many cross-sectional studies. A "total canal seal" afforded by a quality root filling followed by a microbial-tight permanent restoration will secure the periapical health of a well root treated tooth.

Conclusions

- The primary aim of root canal treatment is to eliminate, prevent the recurrence of and exclude new infection from the root canal system.
- Endodontic failures are mainly due to deficiencies or the inability to achieve the primary aim of treatment.
- The objectives of retreatment are to address these inadequacies by gaining access, recleaning, reshaping, redisinfecting and refilling the root canal system, and then re restoring the tooth, so as to achieve and preserve periapical health.
- Although it may not be part of routine retreatment management, unresponsive cases may benefit from microbial sampling to devise an individualised antimicrobial regime. Unfortunately, this is not normally feasible in general practice.

Further Reading

Chong BS, Pitt Ford TR. The role of intracanal medication in root canal treatment. Int Endod J 1992;25:97-106.

Clarkson RM, Moule AJ. Sodium hypochlorite and its use as an endodontic irrigant. Aust Dent J 1998;43:250-256.

Fava LRG, Saunders WP. Calcium hydroxide pastes: classification and clinical indications. Int Endod J 1999;32:257-282.

Hülsmann M, Heckendorff M, Lennon A. Chelating agents in root canal treatment: mode of action and indications for their use. Int Endod J 2003;36:810-830.

Pinheiro ET, Gomes BPFA, Ferraz CCR, et al. Microorganisms from canals of root-filled teeth with periapical lesions. Int Endod J 2003;36:1-11.

Siqueira Jr JF, Lopes HP. Mechanisms of antimicrobial activity of calcium hydroxide: a critical review. Int Endod J 1999;32:361-369.

Sundqvist G, Figdor D, Persson S, Sjögren U. Microbiologic analysis of teeth with failed endodontic treatment and the outcome of conservative re-treatment. Oral Surg Oral Med Oral Pathol Oral Radiol Endod 1998;85:86-93.

Torabinejad M, Handysides R, Khademi AA, Bakland LK. Clinical implications of the smear layer in endodontics: A review. Oral Surg Oral Med Oral Pathol Oral Radiol Endod 2002;94:281-293.

Chapter 5

Disassembling the Coronal Restoration

Aim

To outline techniques required to disassemble coronal restorations, including post removal, and gain entry for non-surgical retreatment.

Outcome

At the end of this chapter, the practitioner should be familiar with techniques to remove coronal restorations and safely remove a variety of post systems.

Introduction

Coronal access is required to enable non-surgical retreatment of an endodontic failure. The methods involved are dependent on the nature and quality of the coronal restoration, some of which may be retained while others may need to be removed completely.

Coronal Restoration

When planning access for retreatment, it is tempting to try and preserve an existing coronal restoration especially if it is:

- technically and aesthetically adequate
- relatively new
- replacement may be costly.

Directly placed intracoronal restorations present no problems, as replacement is relatively easy and inexpensive. If a crown or bridge is present, however, and it may be removed without any damage to the restoration and underlying tooth structure then its preservation may be acceptable. Unfortunately, this is often not possible so it is prudent not to make promises to patients before embarking on treatment.

The desire to preserve a coronal restoration should not be at the expense of having to compromise the requirements of satisfactory access, namely to:

- unroof the entire pulp chamber
- enable an unobstructed view of the canal entrances
- allow instruments to negotiate canals unimpeded
- help retain a temporary restoration.

It is pointless to try and preserve an existing restoration if it jeopardises retreatment; the consequences of retaining a coronal restoration may be great if, because of restricted access, a technical error such as perforation occurs or effective infection control is not achieved.

If the existing coronal restoration requires replacement, there is no need to consider its retention, and the restoration may be removed. The advantages of removing coronal restorations for retreatment, include:

- revealing the state of the underlying tooth structure (Fig 5-1)
- improved vision for the removal of hidden caries
- elimination of covert microleakage
- meticulous inspection for any suspected cracks and fractures
- excellent access for the identification of missed canals.

Whatever the decision, if it is likely that an existing coronal restoration will be damaged, destroyed or need to be removed, then the patient should be advised accordingly, before commencement of retreatment. Patients are more accepting of the need to remove a crown or bridge for retreatment if they are given prior warning.

Factors to consider when deciding whether to retain or remove the coronal restoration are summarised in Fig 5-2.

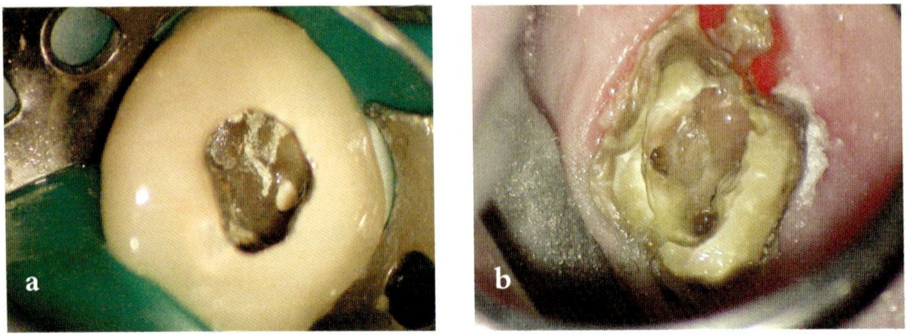

Fig 5-1 Advantage of removing the coronal restoration. (a) Occlusal access cavity in crown. (b) The real picture when the crown is removed!

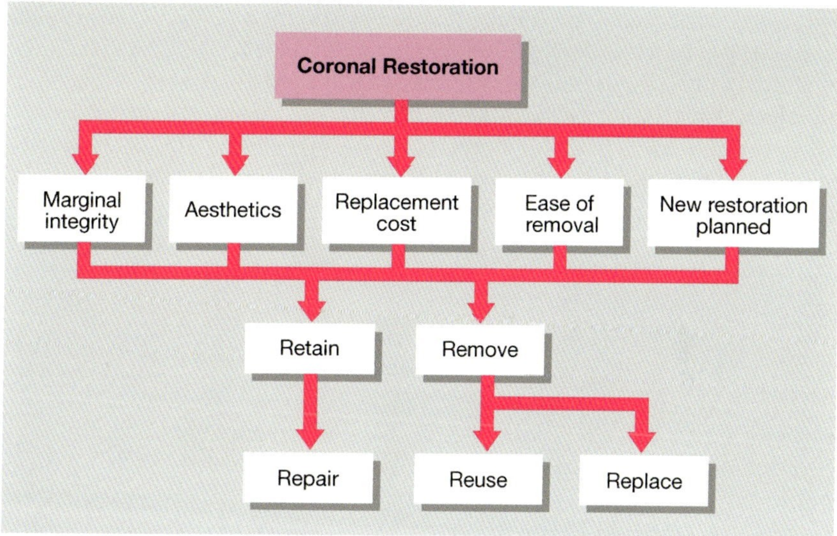

Fig 5-2 Factors to consider when deciding whether to retain or remove the coronal restoration.

Coronal Restoration Removal

Before the coronal restoration is removed, it is crucial to plan the provisional restoration. This may entail taking an impression for chairside fabrication of a temporary restoration or arranging for a laboratory-made temporary replacement. If the tooth is badly broken down, it should be restored beforehand, to protect the remaining tooth tissue and to prevent coronal leakage. A new filling, an orthodontic or copper band or possibly a temporary crown may be needed. For decoronated anterior teeth, an overdenture may be the preferred option, avoiding the risk of cement failure and leakage associated with multiple temporary post crowns.

Crowns and bridges may be removed with a variety of devices; some of which may damage the restoration in the process.

Grasping forceps

Haemostats, some tungsten carbide-tipped, and extraction forceps, such as upper anteriors (Ash 1 & 113, Dentsply Ash Instruments, Weybridge, Surrey, UK) and upper roots pattern (Ash 76 & 76N) may all be used. Great care must be exercised as the haemostat or forceps may slip, especially on porcelain surfaces on which it is difficult to gain good purchase; the porcelain may also break or fracture teeth.

There are also a number of dedicated crown and bridge removal devices on the market (e.g. Carl Martin, Solingen, Germany) (Fig 5-3). The jaws of these grasping devices may have plastic or rubber inserts (Fig 5-4), which may be coated with adhesive or emery powder to prevent slippage, allowing the necessary axial force to be applied more effectively. The action is essentially a pull with some gentle rotation. Care should be taken to avoid injuring adjacent and opposing teeth.

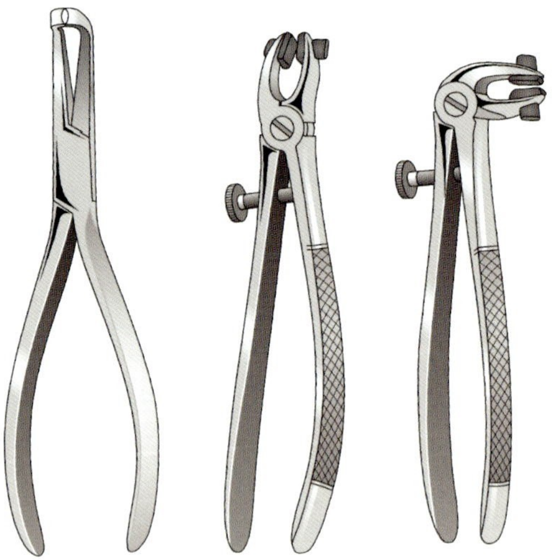

Fig 5-3 Examples of crown removal devices.

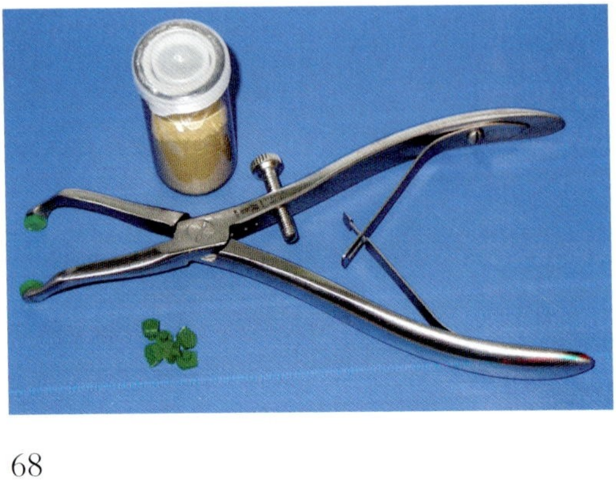

Fig 5-4 Crown and bridge forceps with plastic jaw inserts and adhesive powder in bottle meant for improving grip.

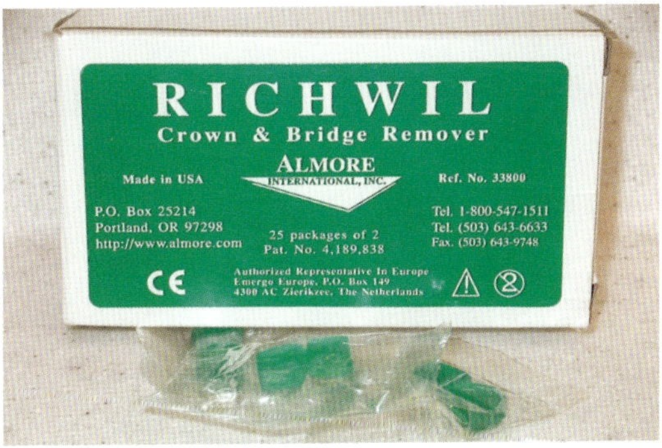

Fig 5-5 Richwil crown and bridge remover.

"Sticky sweet" method
The Richwil crown and bridge remover (Almore International Inc., Portland, OR, USA) (Fig 5-5) is a block of water-soluble, pliable resin, not unlike a sticky sweet. It is first softened in hot water (≈ 63°C) for 1–2 min, removed and excess moisture blotted off. As a precaution, it may be tied with a length of dental floss to aid retrieval in case of accidental ingestion or aspiration. The conditioned resin block is then placed on the restoration to be removed and firm digital pressure applied until it adheres. Next, the patient is asked to bite down, compressing the resin block to two-thirds of its original thickness. Holding this position, the resin block is cooled by spraying with cold water. The patient is then asked to open quickly, generating sufficient force to loosen and lift the restoration. Although marketed as a non-traumatic method, this technique is often not very effective and carries the risk of damaging the opposing tooth or dislodging its restoration. Therefore, always look at the state of the opposing tooth and restoration before using this method!

Levering instruments
A hole of an appropriate size is first made through the occlusal surface of a crown before inserting a straight excavator or Mitchell's trimmer to lever it off. Again, care must be exercised – in particular, with porcelain fused to metal crowns, as the porcelain is likely to break off, even if only a gentle force is applied.

Wedging devices
A slot is cut in the crown using the side of a long-shank tapered bur. This slot is usually cut on the buccal and sometimes extending onto the occlusal

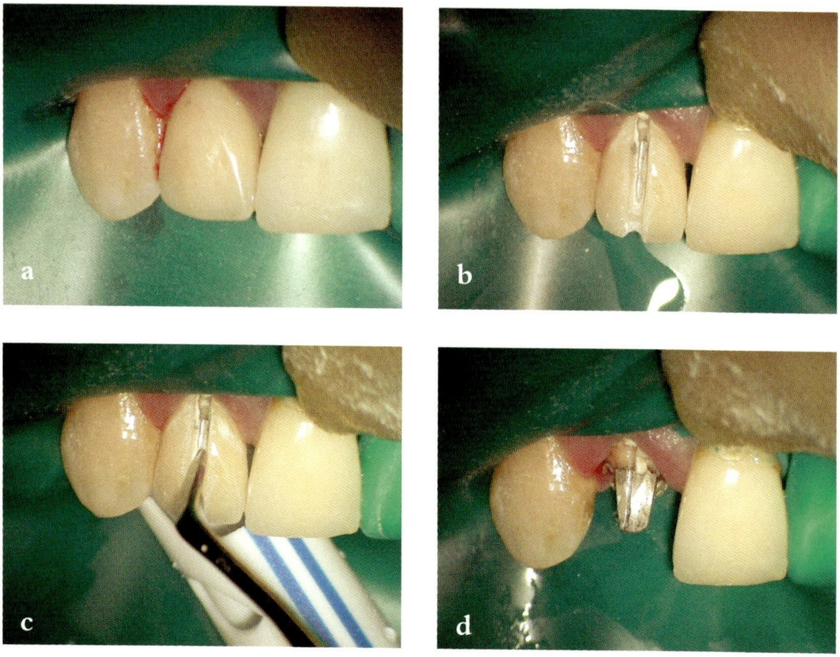

Fig 5-6 Crown removal sequence. (a) A porcelain bonded to metal crown on the lateral incisor. (b) A slot is cut into the crown. (c) A modified flat plastic instrument is used to loosen and wedge the crown apart. (d) The crown successfully removed.

surface of the crown. The cut should be made right through at the gingival margin of the restoration and into the cement lute (Fig 5-6a, b). Generally, diamond burs are best used to cut porcelain and tungsten carbide burs for metal. Special "Transmetal" burs (Dentsply, Weybridge, Surrey, UK) for sectioning metal crowns are also available.

A flat plastic instrument, straight Warwick James or Coupland elevator, modified by flattening the edge (Fig 5-7), is then inserted into the slot to wedge the crown apart (Fig 5-6c), "peeling" it off the tooth (Fig 5-6d). Specially designed crown splitters/separators are also available (Carl Martin, Solingen, Germany) (Fig 5-8) for this purpose.

Tapping and pneumatic tools

A straight chisel and a mallet may be used to tap off a crown. Other devices (Fig 5-9), some spring-loaded, allow the application of tapping forces to

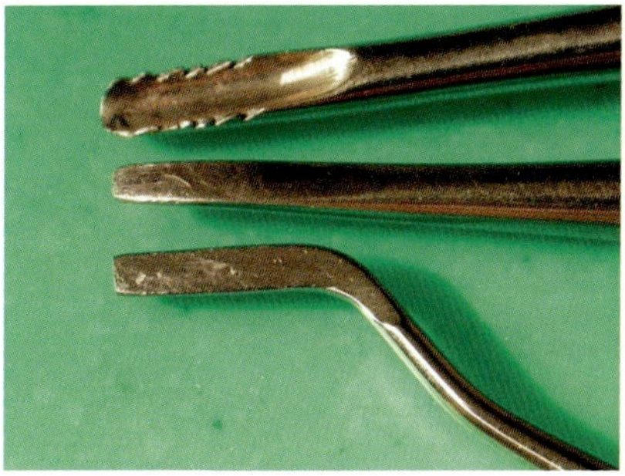

Fig 5-7 Modified instruments used as wedging devices.

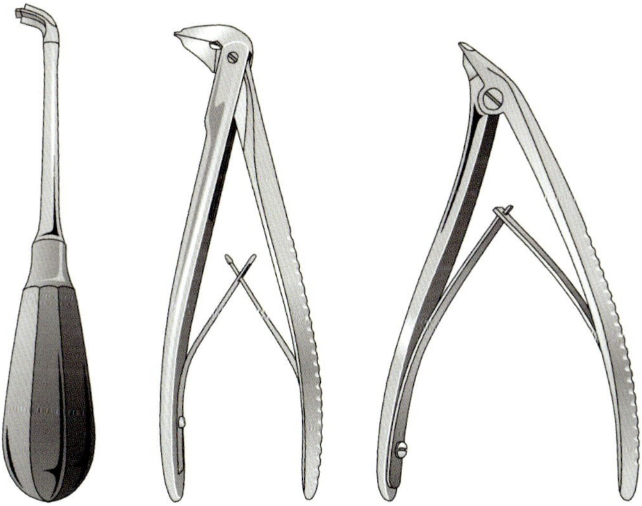

Fig 5-8 Specially designed crown splitters and separators.

loosen the crown. It is often difficult, however, to "hook" well-fitting restorations and apply sufficient force to dislodge the restoration. Bridges can usually be engaged in their embrasures.

The KaVo Coronaflex 2005 device (KaVo Dental Ltd., Amersham, Buckinghamshire, UK) (Fig 5-10) works by delivering a pneumatically generated force at high velocity along the long axis of the tooth, minimising the risk of tooth fracture. Crowns and bridges removed successfully using this

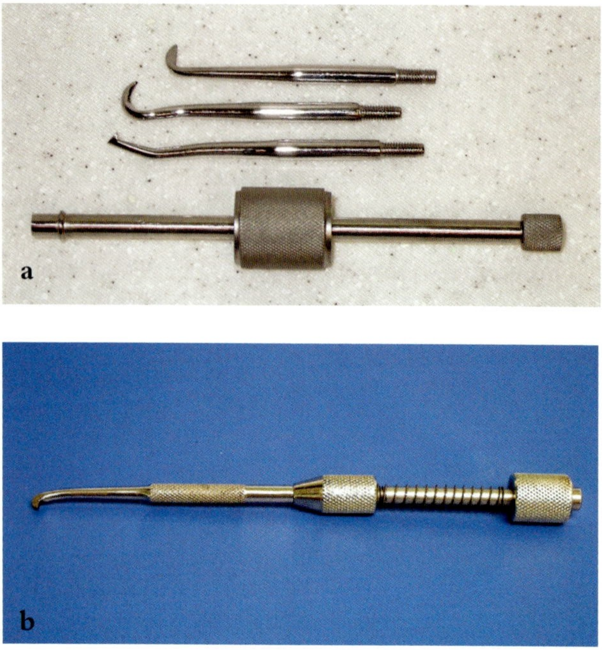

Fig 5-9 Crown and bridge removal tapping devices. (a) Weighted. (b) Spring-loaded.

method can be reused and recemented but there can be no pretreatment guarantees. If the restoration needs to be removed for successful retreatment, this must be the overriding consideration even if the restoration has to be sacrificed in the process.

Ultrasound

Ultrasound may be applied to cast metal crowns and bridges to disrupt the cement lute and act as an adjunct to facilitate removal. Powerful piezo-electric units have many advantages for this purpose and all other dismantling applications. If a restoration with a porcelain surface is to be preserved, for possible reuse, ultrasound should not be applied to it, as the porcelain is almost certain to fracture.

Occlusal Access

If a restoration is to be preserved, the alternative, low-risk option is to make an occlusal access cavity as would be prepared in an intact tooth. There is a variety of burs available for preparing an occlusal access cavity (Fig 5-11). Intracoronal plastic restorations of tooth- and non-tooth-coloured filling materials may be penetrated using high-speed diamond or tungsten carbide burs.

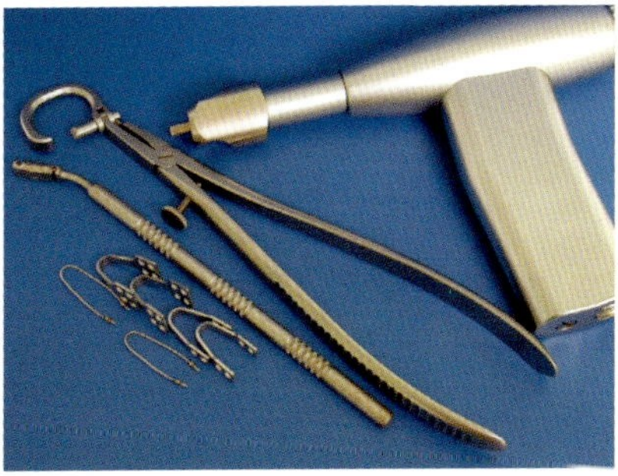

Fig 5-10 KaVo Coronaflex 2005 pneumatic crown and bridge remover.

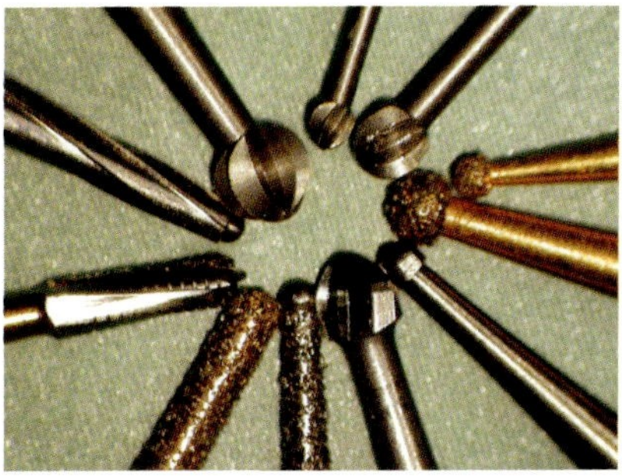

Fig 5-11 Selection of diamond, tungsten carbide and stainless steel burs for achieving occlusal access.

For cast metal restorations, including inlays, high-speed diamond or tungsten carbide burs are appropriate, while diamond burs are needed to cut through porcelain. There is likely to be a core underneath cast restorations. If the core is cast metal, then the overlying restoration will usually have to be removed and its preservation is not possible. If the core consists of either tooth- or non-tooth-coloured filling materials, high-speed diamond or tungsten carbide burs may be used for gross cutting, followed by slow-speed burs, if required, to deal with any remnants of restorative material. Ultrasound is a safe alternative – in particular, when removing material over the furcal floor and around canal orifices. Extra care should be exercised to avoid perforation when removing tooth-coloured filling materials, which are difficult to differentiate from dentine. To help distinguish between the filling material and dentine, an endodontic explorer and magnification may be used; the explorer is abraded by resin composite leaving a grey mark.

Removal of Posts

Posts can be of different compositions and configurations (Fig 5-12) and this will dictate their ease of removal (see Chapter 3, Table 3-1). They may be :

- preformed or custom-made
- parallel-sided or tapered
- smooth-sided, serrated or threaded.

Manufactured from:

- cast metallic alloy - precious or non-precious

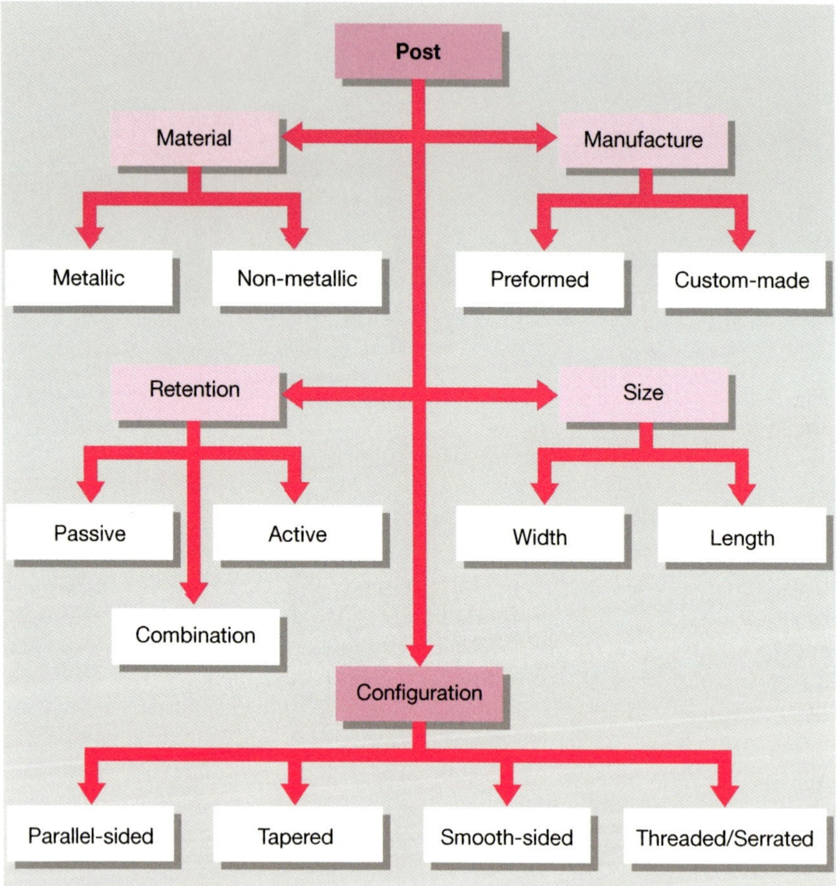

Fig 5-12 Posts can be of different compositions and configurations.

- various metal alloys, if preformed
- non-metallic materials (e.g. carbon fibre, glass or quartz fibres in a composite matrix).

The retention may be achieved:

- passively with luting cement - conventional (e.g. zinc phosphate) or adhesive (e.g. a glass-ionomer) cement
- actively by mechanically engaging the dentine
- with a combination of both.

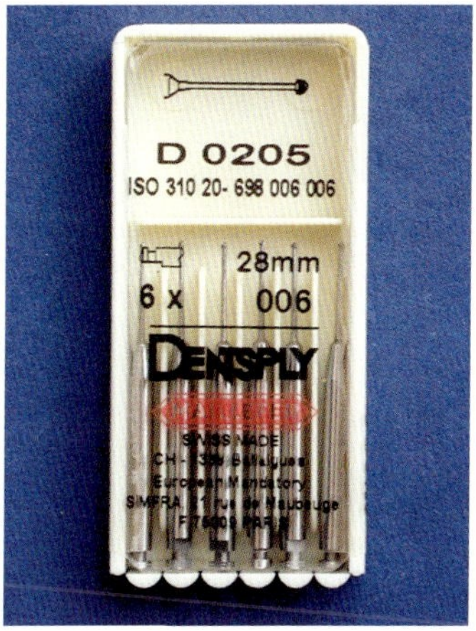

Fig 5-13 Special LN (long neck) round ISO size 006 burs.

Non-metallic posts, such as those made of carbon fibre, glass or quartz fibres in a resin matrix, may be simply drilled out using special burs from the corresponding post remover kit. Alternatively, long neck round ISO size 006 burs (D205 LN bur, Dentsply Maillefer, Ballaigues, Switzerland) (Fig 5-13) and Peeso drills may be used. With carbon fibre posts, a channel is first made down the middle of the post, followed by successively larger sizes of Peeso drills until all the post is removed.

When metallic posts have to be removed, the procedure involves various stages:

Uncover the Post

Remove the coronal restoration

Having decided on the form of temporary restoration and following any necessary preoperative impression, the coronal restoration covering the post and core is first removed (Fig 5-14a, b).

Remove encasing restorative material and cement

With preformed posts, the restorative materials forming the core and encasing the post must be removed. With a cast post and core, the core should be separated from the root face seat by carefully removing dentine/cement at this interface using, for example, a LN bur or ultrasound. The post and core should also be freed from any "ferrule effect" by removing any encircling metal collar using a small metal-cutting round bur (Fig 5-14c).

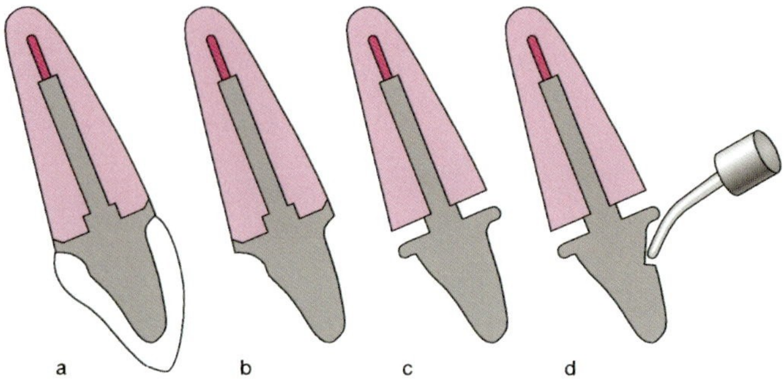

Fig 5-14 Disassembling a coronal restoration. (a) Post crown. (b) Crown removed, core uncovered. (c) Encircling metal collar removed. (d) Rest seat, for the ultrasonic tip, cut into core.

Loosen and Extract the Post

There are then a number of ways of loosening and removing posts:

Use of a bur

If the post is fairly short (5 mm or less), and of a small diameter, it may be possible to drill a channel around the post (Fig 5-15a), loosening it so that it can be removed. A LN bur (Fig 5-13) is recommended if this method of post removal is chosen. Ultrasound may be applied further to loosen the post after a channel is cut between the post and dentine (Fig 5-15d).

Post removal with the aid of a bur should be undertaken with extreme care. A post should never be drilled out using a high-speed metal cutting bur, which carries unacceptable risks of slippage, with loss of control and the likelihood of severe damage to the tooth and surrounding tissues.

Ultrasound

Ultrasound is the most frequently employed method for post loosening and removal. It is used to disrupt the luting cement retaining the post in the root canal. For this purpose, a piezo-electric machine is more effective because it is capable of generating more power than one driven by magnetostriction. The ultrasonic unit should be set to a higher power setting than that for normal tooth scaling. For maximum effectiveness, a large, flat scaler tip, rather than a sickle-shaped tip (Fig 5-16), should be chosen to deliver the ultrasonic vibrations more effectively to the post. Dedicated ultrasonic tips designed for post removal are also available (Fig 5-17).

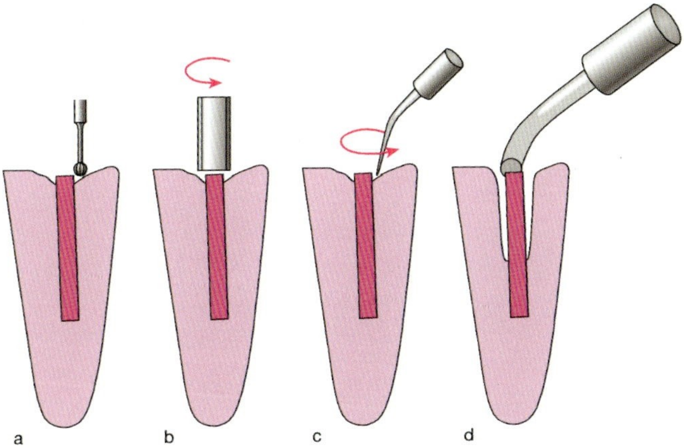

Fig 5-15 Removal of post fractured in canal. Dentine is removed and a channel made around the top of the post using either: (a) a very small bur, (b) a Masserann trepan or (c) a troughing ultrasonic tip. (d) Ultrasound is then applied to loosen the post.

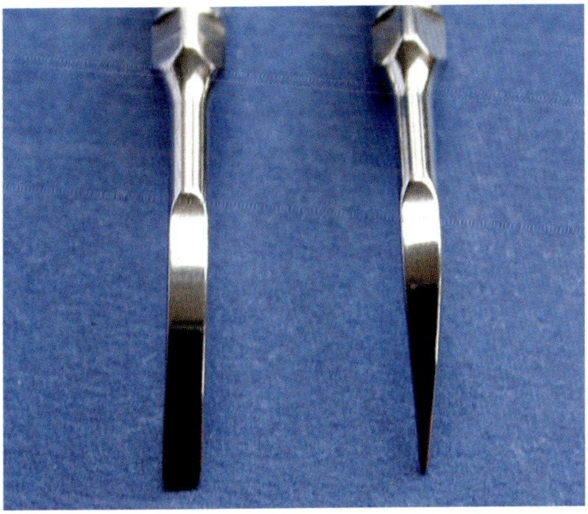

Fig 5-16 Large, flat scaler tip (left) is more efficient in delivering the ultrasonic vibration than a sickle-shaped tip (right).

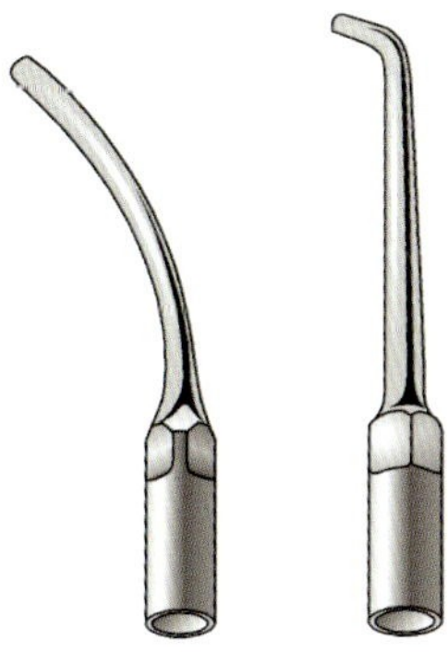

Fig 5-17 Dedicated ultrasonic post removal tips.

In order to prevent the ultrasonic tip from bouncing off the core, a notch may be cut to provide an anchorage point for application of the ultrasonic tip (Fig 5-14d). The ultrasound tip should not be placed perpendicular, but at approximately 30° to the long axis of the core and angled in the coronal direction. The ultrasonic vibrations should be applied in short, intense bursts. In between these bursts, progress should be checked by grasping the post with a suitable instrument such as a pair of upper anterior extraction forceps or haemostat and applying very gentle lateral forces to detect discernible movement. Loosening a post with ultrasound is often a slow process; high expectations of instant results will only be disappointed. Provided there are signs of gradual loosening at each progress check, it is worthwhile continuing. Once the post is loosened sufficiently, it can then be removed. If, however, a post remains solidly in place after a period of, say, 20 min then removal is unlikely to be successful and may have to be abandoned.

If a post is fractured inside a root canal (Fig 5-18a) and ultrasound cannot be applied directly, a fine-beaked forceps, a file or a Masserann extractor (see below) may be used to engage and transmit the ultrasonic vibrations to the post. Alternatively, a trough may be made using a Masserann trepan (Fig 5-15b) or specially designed slim ultrasonic tips (e.g. UT4, SybronEndo, Orange, CA, USA) (Fig 5-15c), some of which are diamond-coated (see Chapter 6, Fig 6-28) or covered with zirconium nitride (Fig 5-19) for better durability. Troughing frees the coronal part of the post, often providing sufficient space between the post and canal wall, to allow the application of ultrasound to loosen the post (Fig 5-15d) which is then removed (Fig 5-18b).

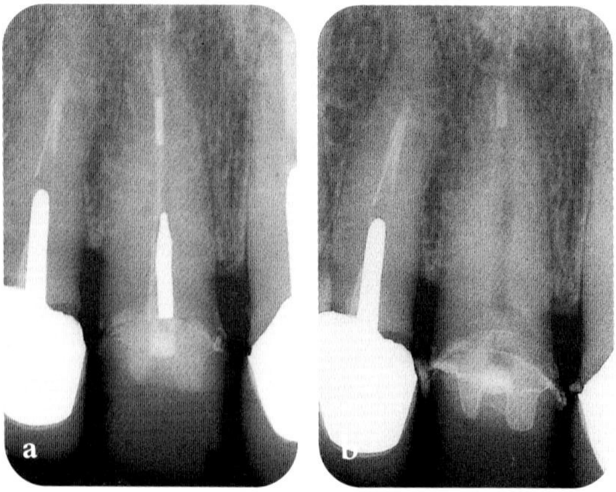

Fig 5-18 Successful removal of a post fractured inside the canal. (a) Pre-op radiograph. (b) Post-op radiograph.

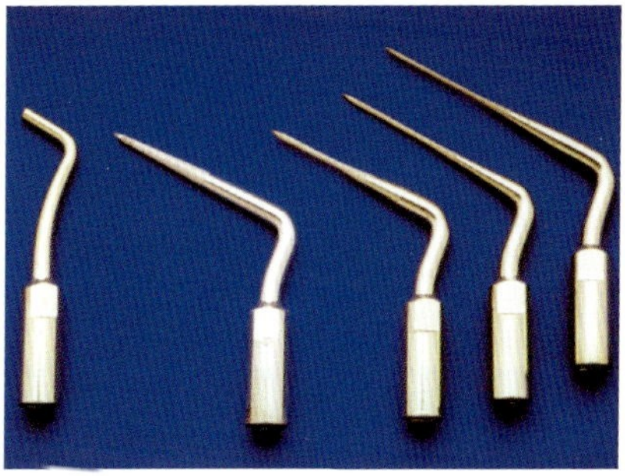

Fig 5-19 Specially designed ultrasonic tips coated with zirconium nitride for durability.

With a screw or threaded post, it is of particular importance to "walk" the ultrasound around the post in an anti-clockwise direction to help loosen and unscrew the post. Sometimes if the screw post is sufficiently loose, it may be possible, and very satisfying, to "spin" it out of the canal using this technique.

With Dentatus (Dentatus AB, Hägersten, Sweden) or Radix Anker (Dentsply, Weybridge, Surrey, UK) screw posts, if the screw head can be uncovered without any damage, the whole post can be unscrewed and removed with a hand wrench from the kit (Fig 5-20). If the top of the screw head is damaged but the rest of the head is mostly intact, a new slot can sometimes be cut for a small screwdriver to unscrew the post (Fig 5-21). Alternatively, cotton-wool (Fig 5-22a) or acrylic resin temporary crown material may be placed into the hollow hand wrench to allow it to engage the damaged screw head without slipping and the post can then be unscrewed (Fig 5-22b). Otherwise, if the screw head is badly damaged, then a pair of fine-beaked forceps or a haemostat may be used to remove the post (Fig 5-23).

Care should always be exercised when attempting screw post removal, non-turning screws should not be forced. It may sometimes be locked with a small tag of filling material, within the canal; ultrasonic vibration may be necessary before further attempts are made. Above all else, be patient and gentle and success will usually follow.

Post removal devices

There are a number of post removal devices on the market. These include the following (Fig 5-24):

- Post Puller (Carl Martin, Solingen, Germany).
- Eggler Post Remover (Automaton-Vertriebs-Gesellschaft, Germany).

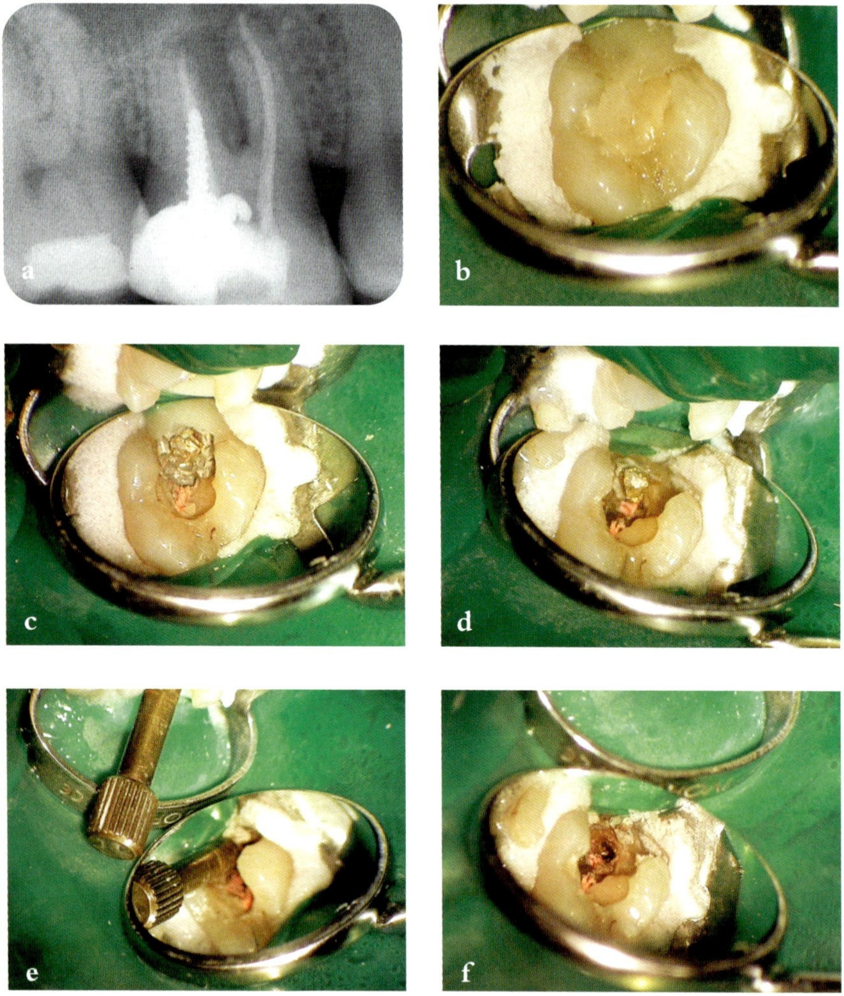

Fig 5-20 Removal of a screw post using a hand wrench. (a) Pre-op radiograph. (b) Tooth isolated with rubber dam. (c) Occlusal access through composite resin restoration. (d) Screw post freed from encasing filling. (e) Hand wrench to engage screw post. (f) Screw post removed.

- Gonon (Thomas) Post Remover (FFDM Pneumat, Bourges Cedex, France).
- Ruddle Post Removal System (SybronEndo, Orange, CA, USA).

All of these devices work like corkscrews creating opposing forces to extract the post from the root canal. Some of the devices are more efficient than others.

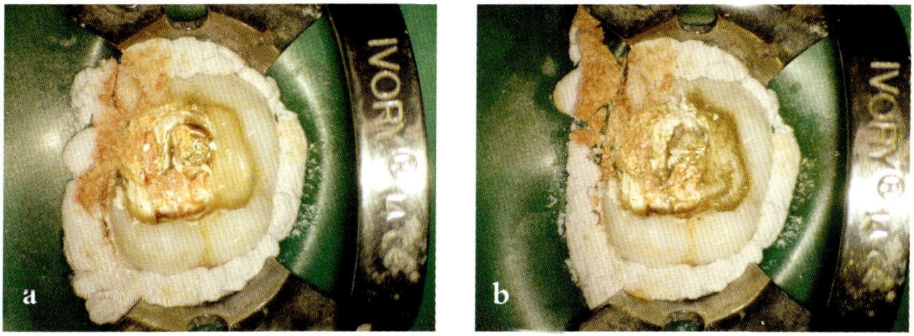

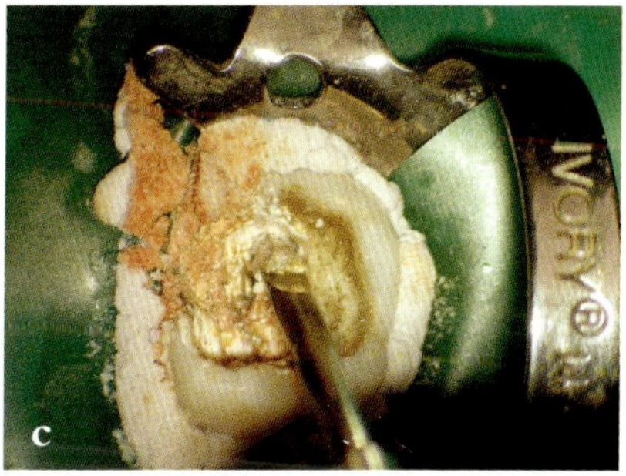

Fig 5-21 Removal of screw post using a screwdriver. (a) Post uncovered. (b) A slot cut into the head of the screw post. (c) A small screwdriver used to unscrew the post.

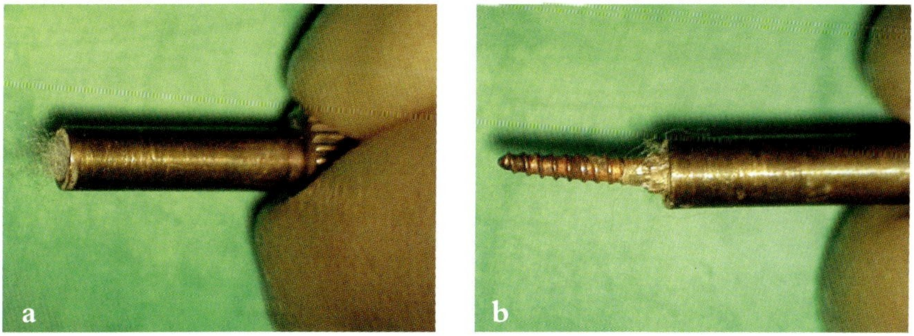

Fig 5-22 If the head of a screw post is damaged (a) cotton wool may be placed into the hollow hand wrench to prevent slippage so that (b) the screw post can then be removed.

With the Eggler and the Post Puller, once the post and core have been exposed, the core is reduced circumferentially to allow the jaws of the device to engage. The two legs of the device are positioned on the root face which may need to be flattened. When the knurled knob is turned, the jaws move coronally, pulling the post out of the canal. Access for these devices may be difficult at

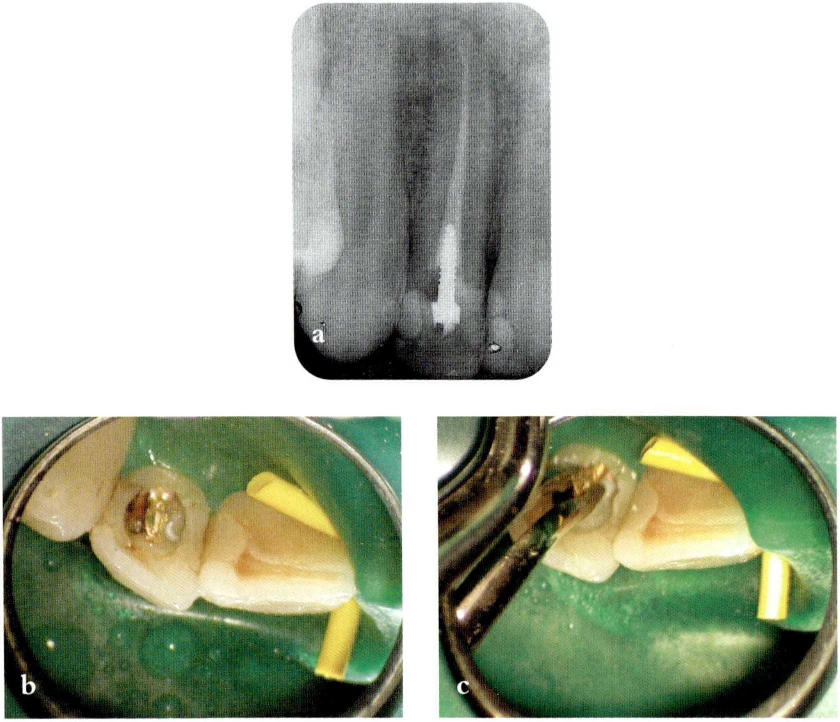

Fig 5-23 Removal of a screw post with a damaged head. (a) Pre-op radiograph. (b) Top of screw post uncovered. (c) Screw post removed using a pair of fine-beaked forceps.

the back of the mouth where the extracting force cannot be applied in an axial direction.

Use of the Gonon post remover requires initial reduction of the core with a long diamond bur prior to creating an inverse countersink with another specially designed bur included in the kit. A trephine is then used to size the core to match a corresponding mandrel, which is tapped onto the core. The extracting pliers, including cushioning washers, are attached, one jaw resting on the root face protected by washers while the other engages the handle of the mandrel. When the knurled knob of the pliers is turned, the jaws move apart, disengaging the post. This is a very powerful, safe and reliable device. The use of the Gonon to remove a fractured post is illustrated in Fig 5-25.

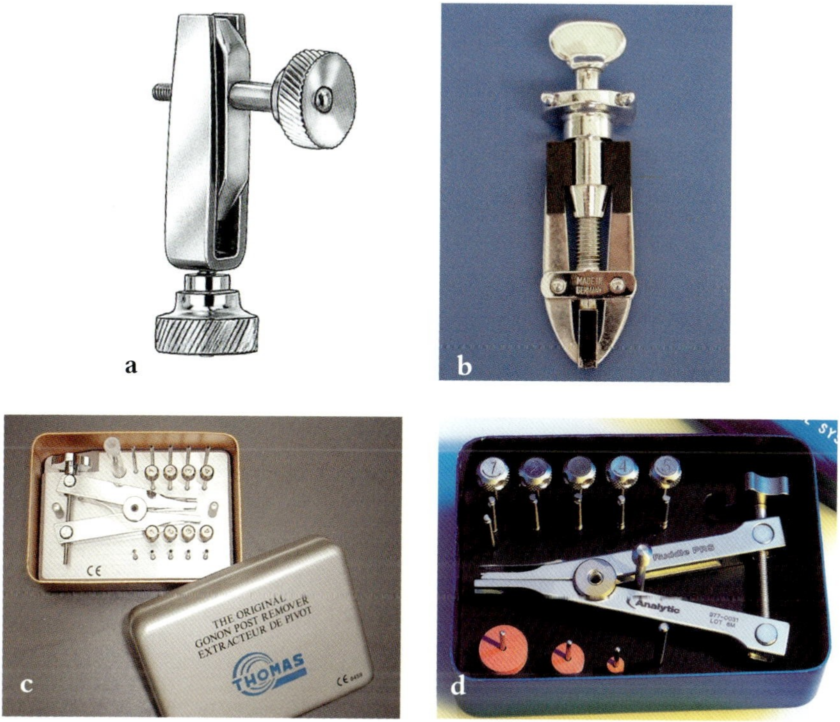

Fig 5-24 Post removal devices: (a) Post Puller. (b) Eggler. (c) Gonon. (d) Ruddle.

The Ruddle Post Removal System is claimed to be an improved version of the Gonon system with a similar mode of action. Both these systems are far more accessible in the posterior region as it can be swivelled into position, to ensure an axial pull on the post.

It should be remembered that threaded or screw posts should not be removed by pulling. The only option may be to try and loosen and unscrew the post. However, if a threaded post is engaged to dentine without an intervening cement lute, there is an unacceptably high risk of root fracture with post pulling devices; surgery may be the only option.

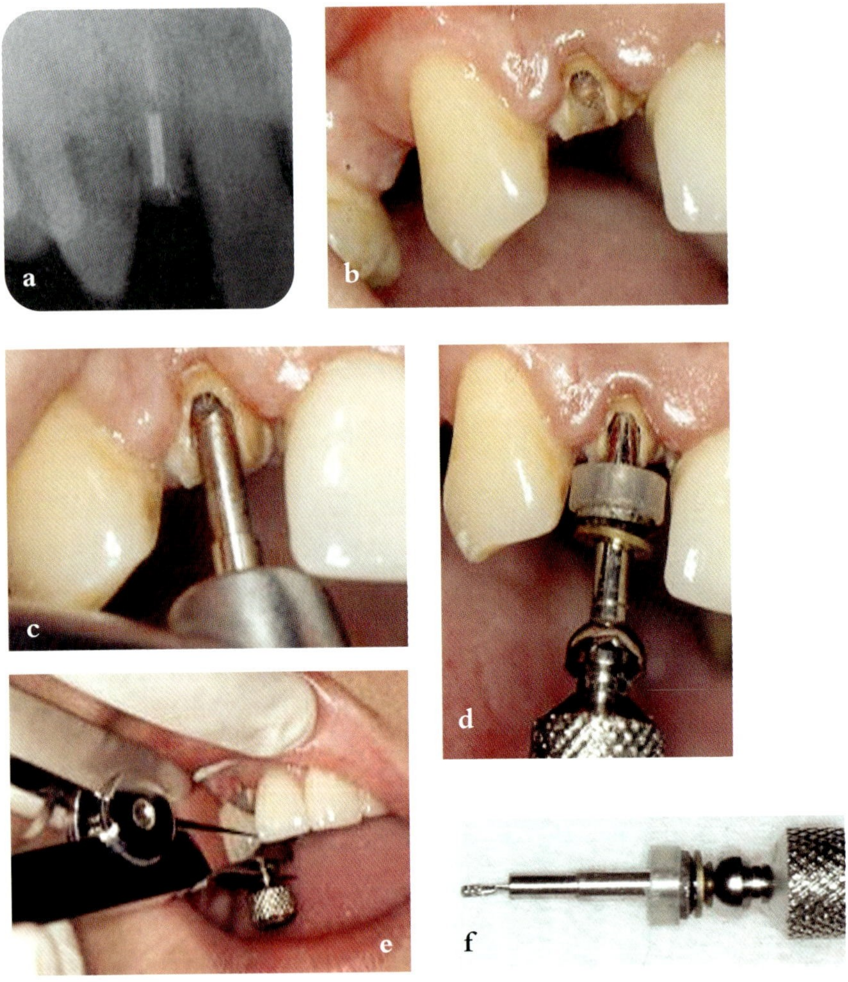

Fig 5-25 Gonon post remover in action. (a) Pre-op radiograph. (b) Clinical view. (c) A trephine bur to size the coronal end of the fractured post. (d) Corresponding mandrel tapped onto the post and washers attached. (e) Extracting pliers engaging mandrel. (f) Post successfully removed. (Courtesy of J. M. Whitworth.)

The Masserann kit

The Masserann technique was devised to remove metallic objects lodged in the root canal. The Masserann kit (Micro-Mega, Besançon, France) (Fig 5-26) consists of:

- Trepans - a series of 14 colour-coded trepans ranging from 1.1–2.4 mm

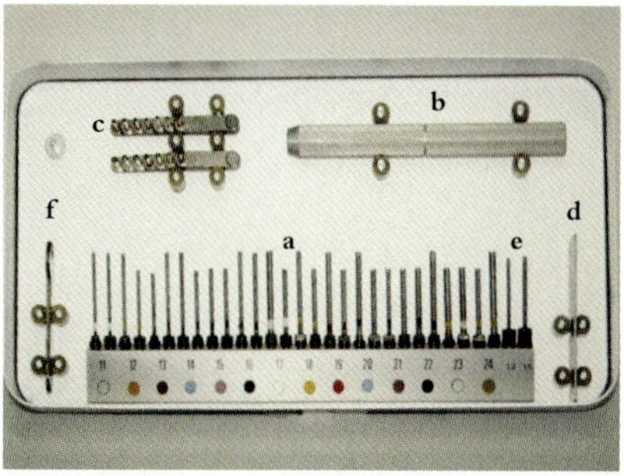

Fig 5-26 Masserann kit. (a) Hollow tubular end-cutting trepans. (b) Handle. (c, d) Gauges. (e) Extractors. (f) A spanner.

in diameter. These trepans are designed for freeing, gripping and extracting large-diameter metallic objects such as posts.
- Extractors - a set of extractors used for smaller-diameter objects such as silver points and instrument fragments.
- Gauges - two sets of tube gauges corresponding to the different sizes of trepans.

The Masserann technique is well documented. In the case of a fractured post (Fig 5-27a, b), the coronal end is first uncovered (Fig 5-27c). With the aid of one of the gauges (Fig 5-27d), a hollow trepan bur is chosen with an internal diameter which corresponds, as closely as possible, to the diameter of the post. The trepan, operated manually or in a speed-reducing handpiece, is rotated in an anticlockwise direction (Fig 5-27e) and advanced slowly to create a trough around the coronal end of the post. This action cuts away at the cement lute, freeing the post and enabling its removal (Fig 5-27f). The Masserann technique is successful where there is adequate access and the root canal is relatively straight, but it results in the sacrifice of root dentine. An effective combination technique, which often preserves apical root dentine, is to alternate between Masserann cutting and ultrasonic vibration. The ultrasound aids post loosening so less dentine removal with the Masserann trepan is necessary.

Meitrac Endo Safety System

The Meitrac system (Hager & Meisinger, Neuss, Germany) (Fig 5-28) is akin to a reduced version of the Masserann. The system consists of trepans and extractors, designed to remove intraradicular obstructions of different diameters:
- Meitrac I – 0.15 to 0.5 mm, for broken instruments
- Meitrac II – 0.5 to 0.9 mm, for silver points
- Meitrac III – 0.9 to 1.5 mm, for posts.

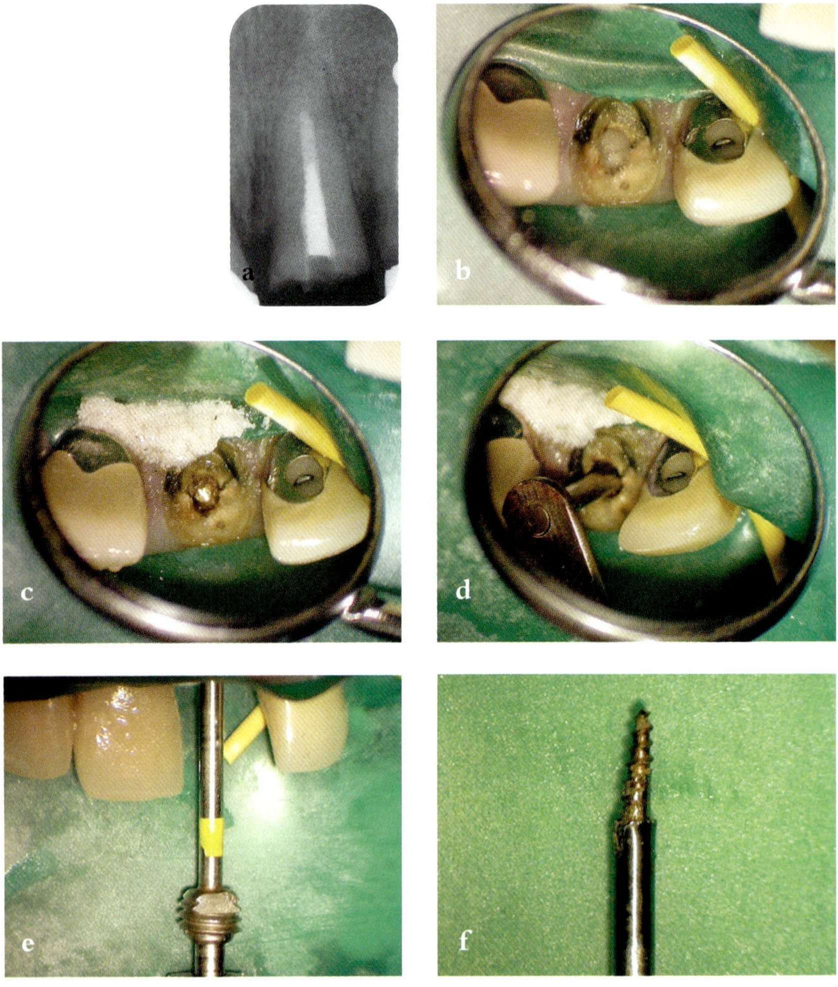

Fig 5-27 Screw post removal using the Masserann kit. (a) Pre-op radiograph. (b) Tooth isolated with rubber dam. (c) Coronal end of screw post uncovered. (d) Gauge used to determine size of Masserann trepan needed. (e) Chosen trepan operated in an anti-clockwise direction. (f) Post removed successfully.

In the Meitrac III range, the diameters of the two trepans match the two extractors (1.2 and 1.5 mm). As with the Masserann system, the trepan to be used is selected according to the diameter of the post. Following use of the trepan, the corresponding extractor is then employed.

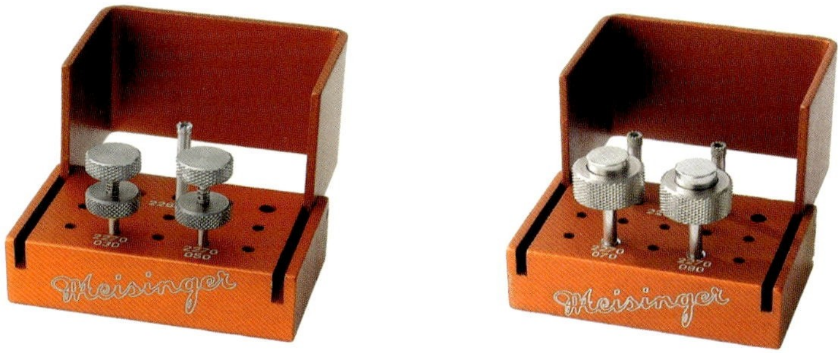

Fig 5-28 Meitrac Endo Safety System.

Post removal used to be regarded as a dangerous procedure often associated with root fracture. As a result, cases requiring post removal were often considered suitable only for surgery. Recent developments, particularly in the use of ultrasound, have made root fracture a rarity, and rapid safe post removal is now the norm rather than the exception.

Conclusions

- Coronal access is required to enable non-surgical retreatment of endodontic failures.
- The patient should be advised preoperatively as to the risk of an existing coronal restoration being damaged, destroyed or requiring removal for non-surgical retreatment.
- Before the coronal restoration is removed, careful consideration must be given to the provision of an interappointment restoration which will protect and seal the tooth.
- The quality and design of an existing restoration tend to dictate the approach to achieve coronal access.
- Ultrasound, typically supplemented by pulling or trephining devices, is the most universally useful method for coronal disassembly.

Further Reading

Castrisos T, Abbott PV. A survey of methods used for post removal in specialist endodontic practice. Int Endod J 2002;35:172-180.

Hauman CHJ, Chandler NP, Purton DG. Factors influencing the removal of posts. Int Endod J 2003:36:687-690.

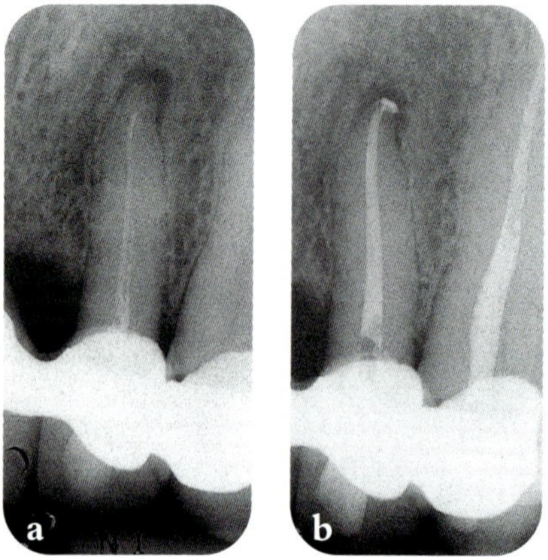

Fig 6-1 A poorly condensed gutta percha root filling is likely to be loose and relatively easy to remove. (a) Pre-op radiograph. (b) Post-op radiograph.

the file is withdrawn, it should pull the gutta percha root filling free of the canal (Fig 6-2). The action is repeated as necessary with successive larger sizes of files until all the gutta percha is removed.

Barbed broaches (Fig 6-3) may be used in the same way, but they should be inserted in a "watch-winding" motion (see Chapter 7, Fig 7-16) as they are made from very soft steel and susceptible to breakage if screwed into the canal.

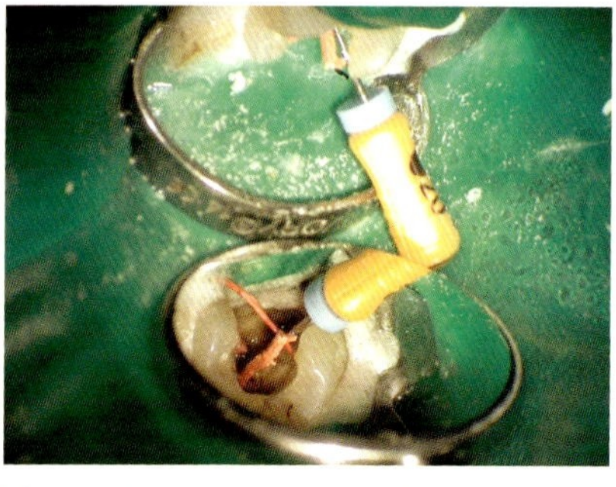

Fig 6-2 Loose gutta percha root filling removed using a Hedstrom file.

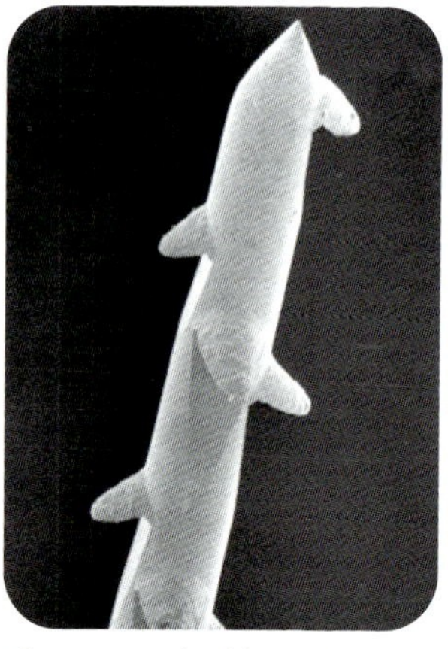

Fig 6-3 Barbed broach (SEM).

Rotary files

A rotary file is chosen so that the cutting flutes will engage the root filling and not the canal walls; when activated, the flutes should "churn" out the root filling. To reduce the risk of rotary file breakage, in particular with small size files, caution should be exercised not to apply excessive apical pressure and to keep within the recommended speed and torque limits of the chosen rotary system.

Ultrasound

Ultrasound may also be used to remove a single cone or poorly condensed gutta percha root filling (Fig 6-4). An ISO size 15 endosonic file is inserted into the root canal. When activated, a combination of irrigation and ultra-

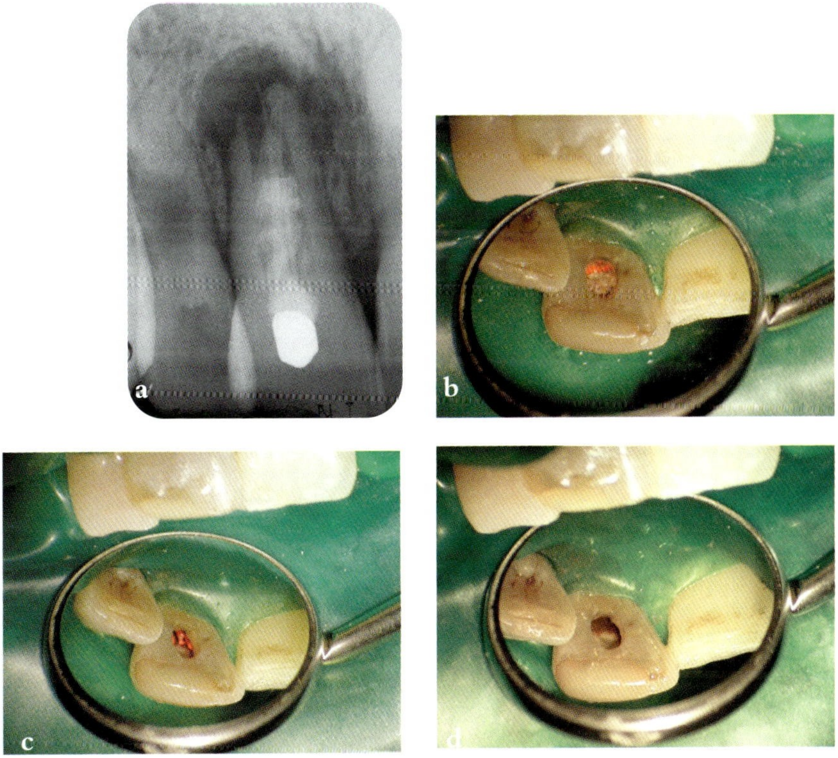

Fig 6-4 Removal of multiple, loose gutta percha cones. (a) Pre-op radiograph. (b) Palatal access cavity. (c) Gutta percha cones uncovered after removal of underlying cement and debris with an ultrasonic scaler. (d) Empty canal after root filling removed using an ultrasonically activated, irrigated file.

sonic vibration will break down the sealer, loosening and allowing the gutta percha to float out. The file must be irrigated rather than run dry. Otherwise, the gutta percha will be plasticized, making it difficult to remove the root filling intact.

Condensed Gutta Percha

A well-condensed gutta percha root filling cannot be removed en masse. It must first be softened with heat or solvents.

Heat

Heat may be applied using:

- old instruments including pluggers and probes or special heat-retentive spreaders and pluggers (e.g. GP2 and GP3 heat carriers, Hu-Friedy, Chicago, IL, USA), which are heated in an open flame (Fig 6-5)
- electrically heated spreaders and pluggers like the "Touch 'n Heat" (SybronEndo, Orange, CA, USA) (Fig 6-6) or System B (see Chapter 4, Fig 4-16).

A Hedstrom file is then used to engage a portion of the heat-softened gutta percha, which is removed when the file is withdrawn. Heat is then reapplied and the procedure repeated until all the material is removed. Heat may also be created when drilling out the gutta percha using:

- Gates-Glidden drills
- long-neck burs
- specially-designed gutta percha removal instruments.

Gates-Glidden drills and long-neck burs are limited by the depth to which they may be used in the canal – in particular, a curved root, where they have to be confined to the straight part of the canal. Gutta percha removal

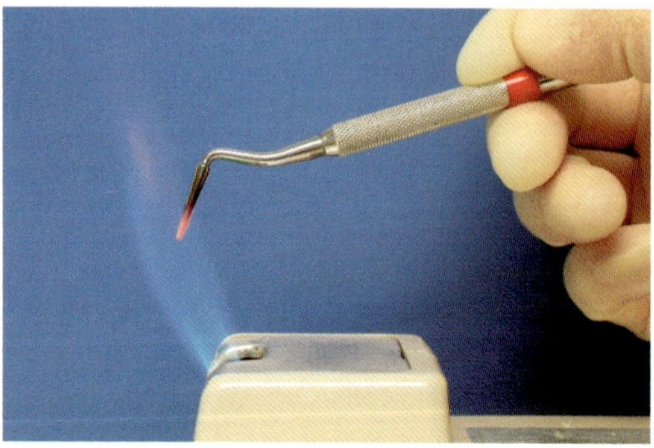

Fig 6-5 Heated plugger used to aid removal of condensed gutta percha root filling.

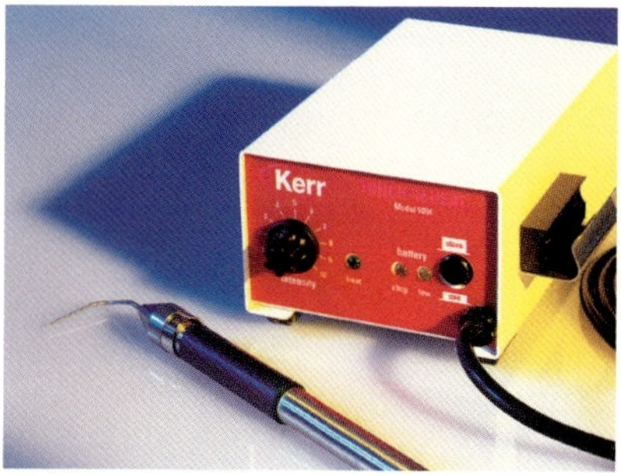

Fig 6-6 "Touch 'n Heat", an electrically-heated spreader device.

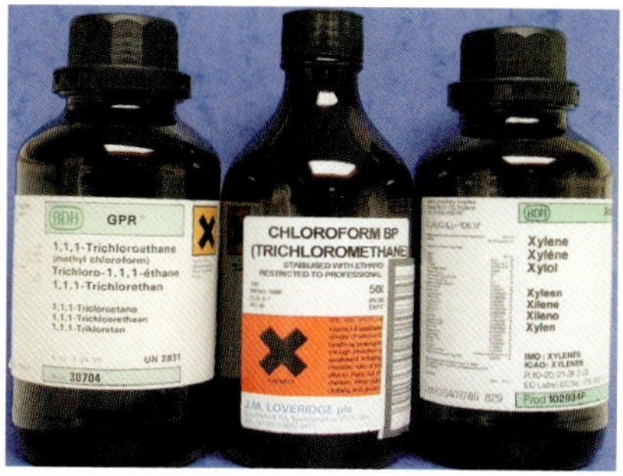

Fig 6-7 Gutta percha solvents.

instruments (e.g. GPX, Brasseler USA, Savannah, GA, USA) are more effective than Gates-Glidden drills or long-neck burs. When operated in a root canal, the frictional heat generated softens the gutta percha which is evacuated coronally by the cutting flutes, operating in an Archimedian screw principle. There is always a risk of fracture when using gutta percha removal instruments. As a result, great care must be exercised, avoiding excessive force and too high a rotational speed. All these instruments may facilitate removal of most of the root filling – however, some gutta percha remnants are inevitable and its removal requires the use of a solvent.

Solvents

The use of solvents particularly deep in the canal is safer and comparably more effective and faster than using heat. Numerous gutta percha solvents (Fig 6-7) have been evaluated, including:

- chloroform
- eucalyptol oil
- xylene (xylol)
- rectified turpentine
- methyl chloroform
- halothane.

These solvents are available from larger pharmacies and laboratory chemical suppliers. Some solvents are more effectiv than others. Chloroform is highly effective and the most popular gutta percha solvent. Concerns have been expressed, however, about its carcinogenic potential, although evidence is limited. Xylene may also be carcinogenic, whilst rectified turpentine, methyl chloroform, and halothane have been suggested as safer alternatives.

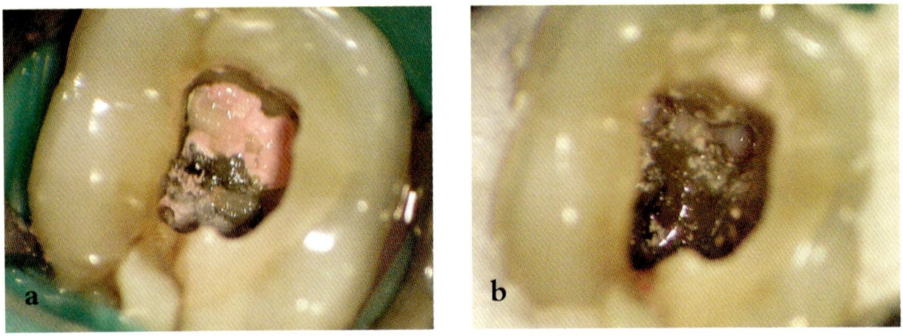

Fig 6-8 Using a solvent to aid removal of condensed gutta percha. (a) Root filling exposed. (b) Gutta percha in coronal part of canals cleared with Gates-Glidden burs and solvent placed in wells created in canal entrances.

For the most efficient use of solvents, the pulp chamber and the coronal part of the canal should be cleared of gutta percha with a Gates-Glidden bur, a NiTi coronal flaring rotary file or a heated instrument, to create a well (Fig 6-8a). If the solvent is placed in the pulp chamber instead of into a well, it will evaporate more quickly because of the greater surface area. In addition, a well permits intimate contact between the solvent and gutta percha.

The chosen solvent is drawn up into a small syringe made of glass, polypropylene, or other materials not affected by the solvent. A 1 mL syringe is ideal for the small volume needed. The well is then filled with solvent (Fig 6-8b), avoiding flooding the pulp chamber since excess solvent will evaporate or run onto the rubber dam which may be dissolved or punctured.

A hand or rotary file is then used to work the solvent into the gutta percha to hasten its dissolution. As the file is rotated gently, advanced and then withdrawn, the softened gutta percha is removed. Gutta percha is wiped off the file with gauze before being reinserted. The process is repeated until most of the gutta percha has been removed. Any residual gutta percha will be eliminated when the canal is reprepared. Alternatively, more solvent may be added to dissolve any remnants and paper points used to soak up the dissolved gutta percha (Fig 6-9). If necessary, a radiograph may be taken to ensure that all previous root filling material has been removed. Gutta percha solvents are tissue irritants and should be used sparingly. Care should also be taken to ensure that solvents are not extruded through the root apex into the periapical tissues by keeping instruments within the canal.

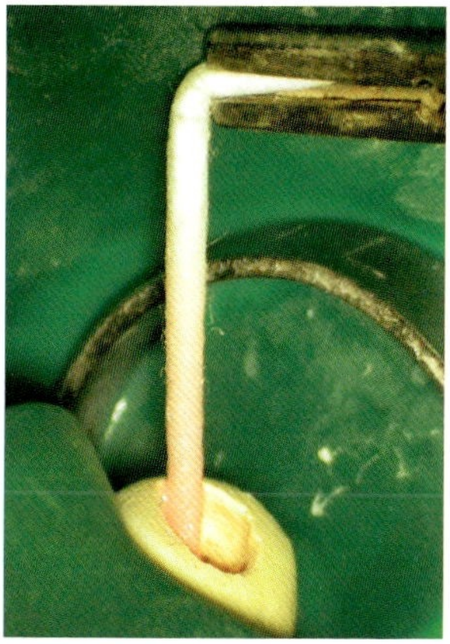

Fig 6-9 Paper points used to soak up dissolved gutta percha remnants.

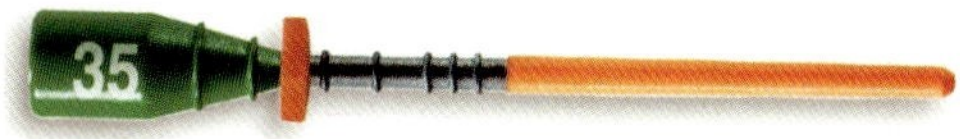

Fig 6-10 Thermafil obturator.

Gutta Percha Carrier Devices

The Thermafil system (Dentsply Maillefer, Ballaigues, Switzerland) is perhaps the best-known example of a gutta percha carrier device. This commercial product originated from a technique of moulding heated gutta percha to a root canal file, which was then warmed and inserted to fill the prepared canal. The coronal excess is removed, leaving the apical part behind in the canal. A major disadvantage of these devices is that a retained obturator is more difficult to remove than gutta percha alone.

The cores of Thermafil obturators were originally made of plastic, titanium or stainless steel – all of which may be encountered. There have, however, been a number of design changes. The latest Thermafil obturators (Fig 6-10) have a 0.04 taper, with a V-shaped cross-section plastic core, which is coated with alpha phase gutta percha. The V-shaped groove is designed to aid removal of the obturators when retreatment is required. Several copycat systems have no such helpful groove.

The best way to remove carrier devices is to use a gutta percha solvent to dissolve the gutta percha coating the carrier. If the carrier is made of:

- metal (Fig 6-11) - once it is exposed and worked loose, it can be treated as a broken instrument (see Chapter 7)
- plastic (Fig 6-12) - once softened with a solvent, the carrier is removed in a similar manner to condensed gutta percha. Alternatively, a Hedstrom file may be used to engage and extract the loosened carrier.

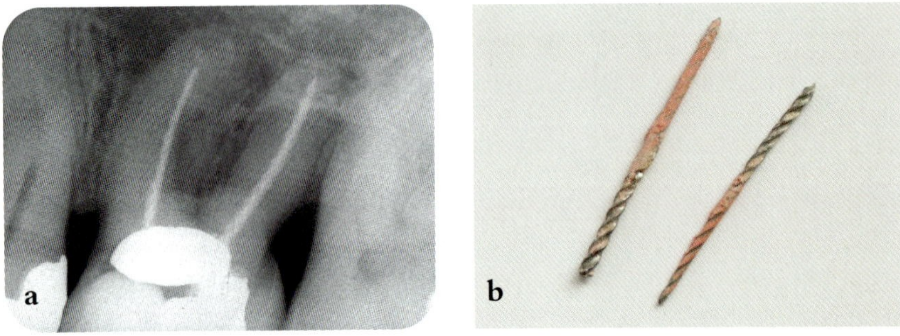

Fig 6-11 Gutta percha carrier devices with metal core. (a) Pre-op radiograph. (b) Removed carriers.

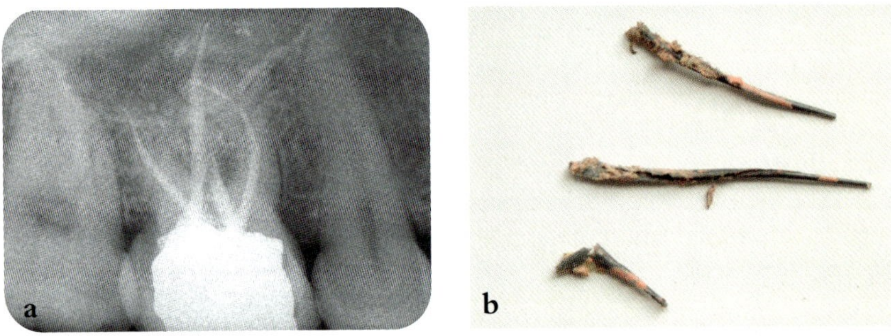

Fig 6-12 Gutta percha carrier devices with plastic core. (a) Pre-op radiograph. (b) Removed carriers.

Removal of Silver Points

Rigid core root filling materials including silver points were once in vogue but are no longer regarded as satisfactory as they do not seal root canals completely. For this reason, they are often seen in cases presenting for retreatment. Silver points (Fig 6-13) are made of relatively soft silver alloys containing 0.1–0.2% of copper and nickel.

When removing silver points, it should also be remembered that their corrosion products are toxic (Fig 6-14). Copious irrigation must therefore be used and great care exercised to ensure corrosion products are not pushed out of the apex as this may provoke undesirable acute consequences. Silver point corrosion products may also cause gingival tattooing (Fig 6-15).

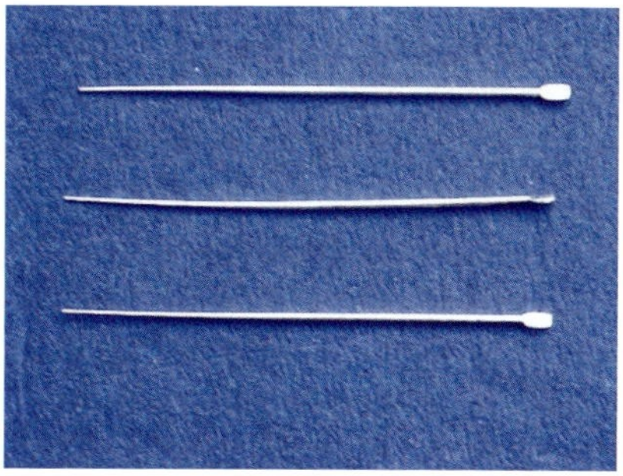

Fig 6-13 Silver points, a rigid core root filling material.

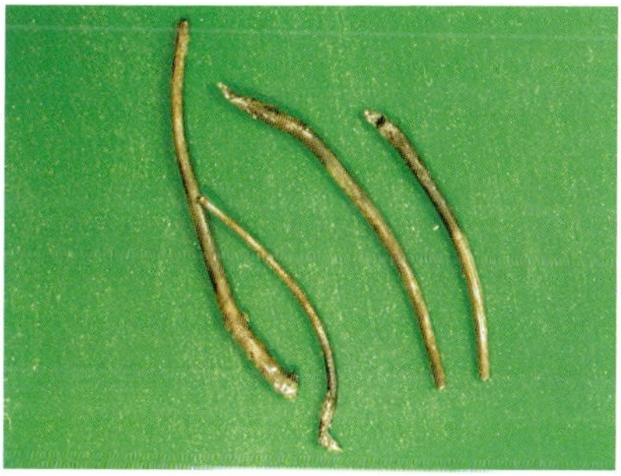

Fig 6-14 Corroded silver points, removed from a tooth.

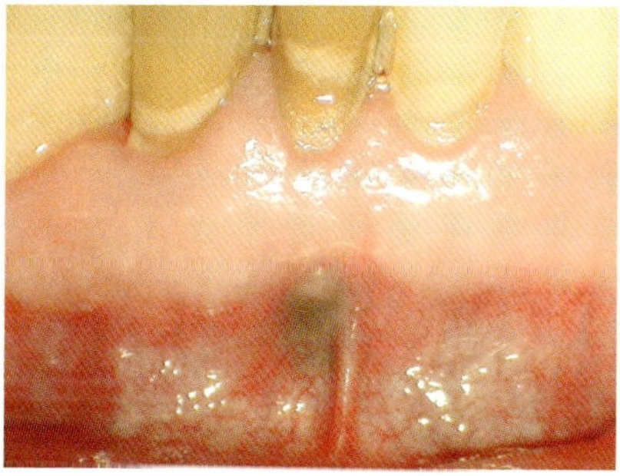

Fig 6-15 Gingival tattooing caused by corrosion products from silver point root filling.

A silver point can usually be removed successfully (Fig 6-16) if it is:

- visible and accessible
- loose
- possible to gain purchase.

Visible and Accessible

Great care must be taken so as not to cut off the coronal end of the silver point, which extends into the pulp chamber. Material surrounding the silver point is best removed gently with an ultrasonic scaler, taking care to avoid touching the silver point directly with the scaler to prevent weakening or breaking off its coronal end. If embedded in amalgam, the coronal ends of silver points may be especially difficult to find; the amalgam should be sectioned carefully with a bur and then removed using ultrasound.

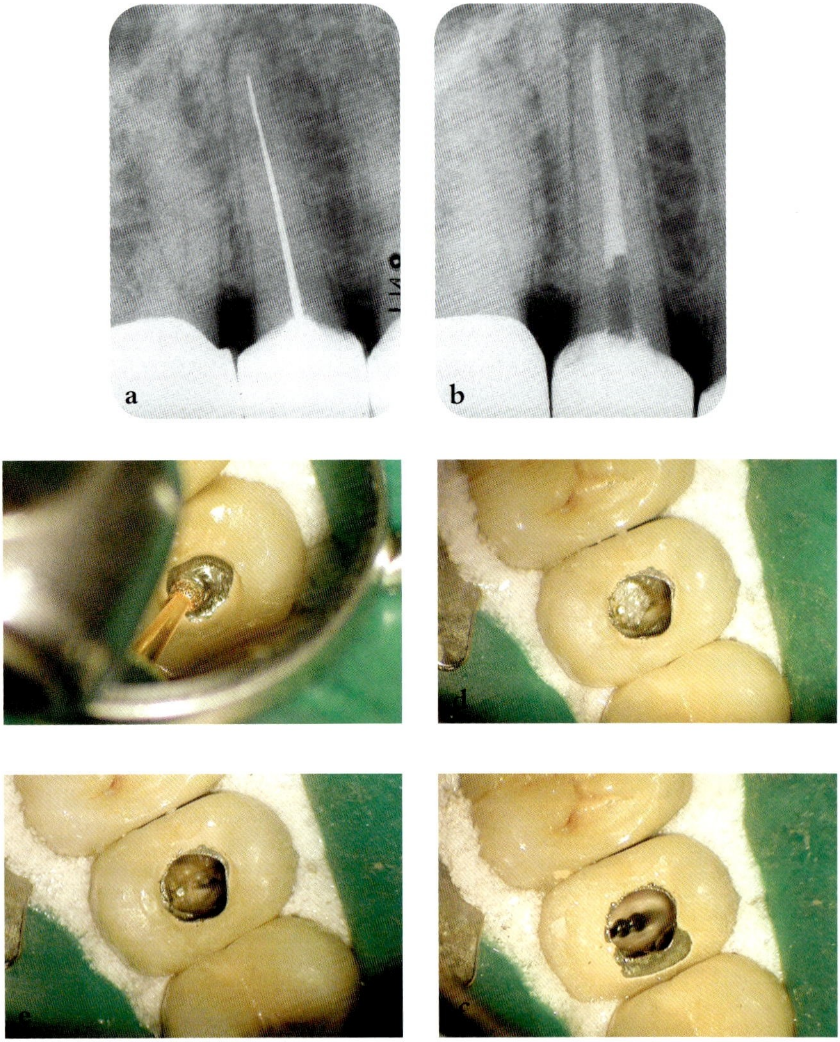

Fig 6-16 Non-surgical retreatment of a silver point root filling. Radiographs (a) pre-op (b) post-op. Procedure: (c) occlusal access through the existing porcelain bonded to metal crown. (d) Silver point visible, encased in amalgam core. (e) Silver point uncovered. (f) Silver point removed, caries and debris cleared to reveal a fin-shaped canal.

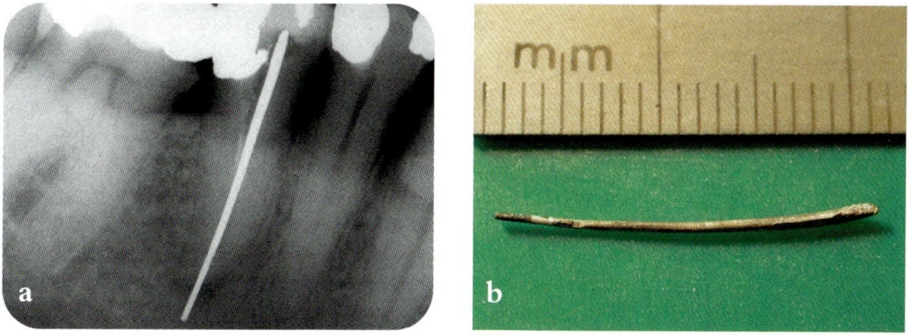

Fig 6-17 Non-surgical retreatment of an overextended silver point root filling. (a) Pre-op radiograph. (b) The removed silver point.

Loose

If the silver point is wedged tightly, it needs to be loosened by removing whatever is encasing it. Dentine, cement or filling material around the coronal portion of the silver point can again be safely removed using ultrasound. Hand, rotary, ultrasonic or sonic files may then be inserted and worked circumferentially to loosen the silver point within the canal. Silver points inserted with resin-based sealers – for example, AH 26 (Dentsply DeTrey-DeDent, Konstanz, Germany) – are very resistant to removal because it is difficult to break the cement lute. A gutta percha solvent may help, but some sealers are very resistant to dissolution. An overextended silver point, wedged in the apical foramen is particularly challenging to remove (Fig 6-17); if all else fails, surgery may be required.

Possible to Gain Purchase

Once loosened and when sufficient length has been uncovered, the coronal end may be grasped and the silver point extracted using a variety of instruments (Fig 6-18) including:

- tweezers
- a fine-beaked haemostat
- Steiglitz forceps (Hu-Friedy, Chicago, IL, USA) (Fig 6-19)
- levered out using a spoon excavator or Caulfield silver point retriever (Miltex Inc., York, PA, USA).

If the exposed coronal end is too short or impossible to grab hold of, then removal may be attempted using one of the following:

- *Hedstrom file* - if there is plenty of space alongside the silver point, a Hedstrom file may be used to engage and extract the silver point. The cutting flutes of the Hedstrom file are particularly effective for this purpose.

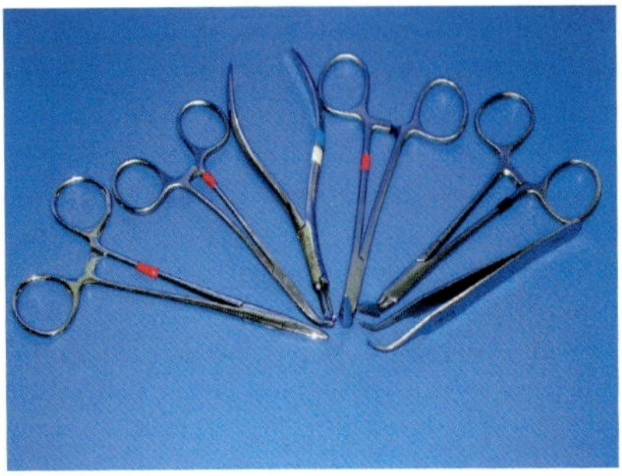

Fig 6-18 Grasping devices for extracting silver points and other retained intracanal objects.

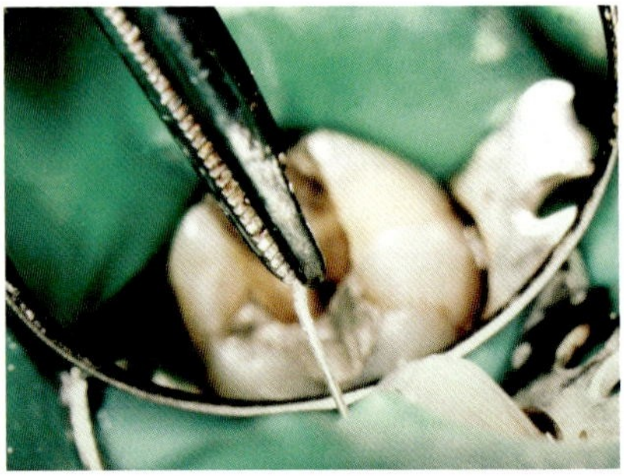

Fig 6-19 Silver point removed with Steiglitz forceps.

- *Braiding technique* (Fig 6-20) - three small (e.g. ISO size 15) Hedstrom files are first worked alongside the silver point. With the files inserted, they are twisted and braided around the silver point to engage it. The silver point is removed when the files are withdrawn together. However, this method of silver point removal is only successful provided there is sufficient space adjacent to the silver point to place multiple files. If incorrectly applied there is the risk of breaking files inside the root canal, compounding the problem.
- *Masserann extractor* (Fig 6-21a) - consists of a hollow tube with a constriction, which is placed over the coronal end of the silver point. A stylet is then inserted into the hollow tube to trap the silver point against the constriction - a minimum of 3 mm is needed for effective purchase. When the extractor is removed, the silver point is then pulled out (Fig 6-21b).
- *Meitrac Endo Safety System* (see Chapters 5 and 7) - the Meitrac II is designed for silver point removal. It consists of a trepan (0.21 mm diameter) and two extractors (0.7 or 0.9 mm diameter). The trepan may be used to create a trough around the top of the silver point and an extractor, which is spring-loaded, is then chosen to engage and remove the silver point. Again, a minimum of 3 mm is needed for effective purchase.
- *Ultrasound and sonic devices* - an ISO size 15 ultrasonically or sonically-energised file, combined with high-volume irrigation, may be used to float out a silver point. Provided the silver point is of a relatively small size and loose, this technique may be effective.
- *Cancellier extractor* (SybronEndo, Orange, CA, USA) - these extractors (Fig 6-22) are a set of hollow tubes, which fit into a handle; the assembly resembling a hollow plugger. The appropriate size extractor is chosen to fit

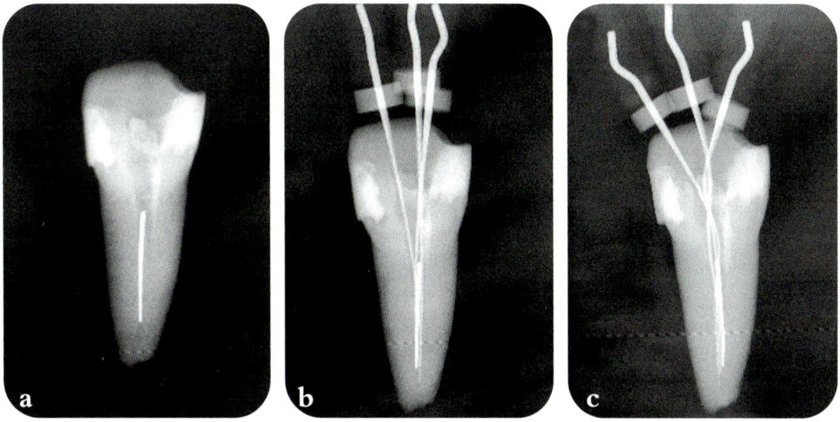

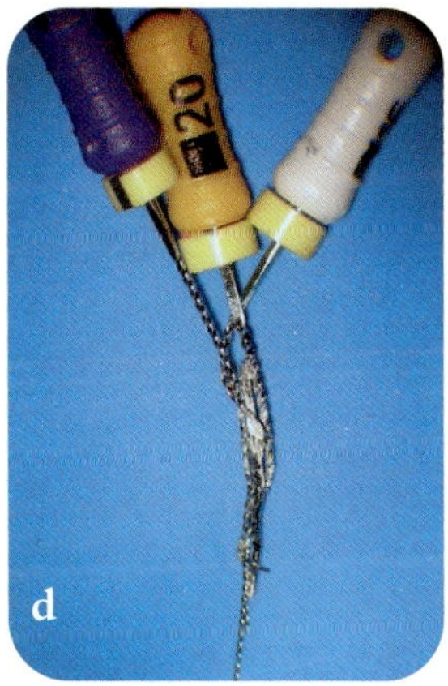

Fig 6-20 Silver point removal using the braiding technique. (a) Silver point root filling. (b) Three small size files inserted alongside the silver point. (c) Files twisted together to engage silver point. (d) Silver point extracted when files withdrawn together.

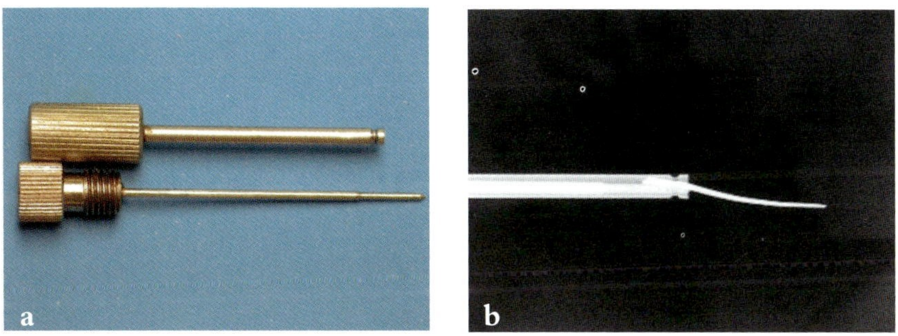

Fig 6-21 Masserann extractor. (a) A hollow tube with a constriction (top) and a stylet (bottom). (b) The stylet locks the silver point against the constriction of the extractor.

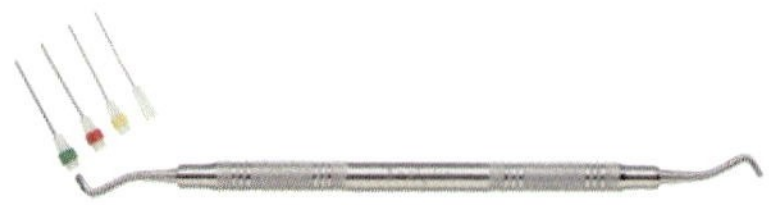

Fig 6-22 Cancellier extractor.

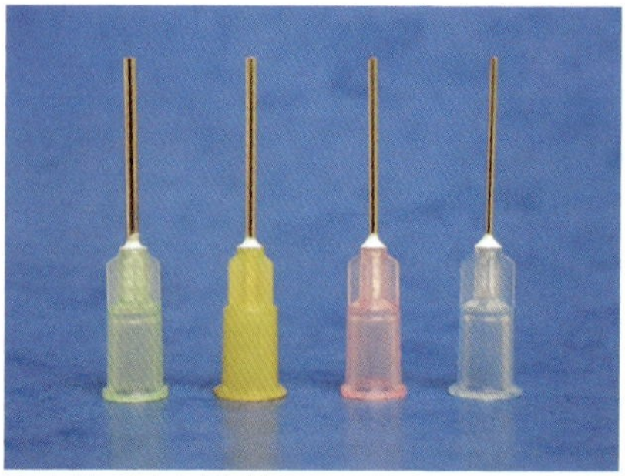

Fig 6-23 Endo-Eze tips (left to right): 18, 19, 20, 22 gauge.

closely over the silver point. A drop of cyanoacrylate glue is placed into the hollow end of the extractor so that it adheres when fitted over the silver point. A drop of acrylic monomer liquid can then be used to accelerate the setting of the cyanoacrylate glue and the silver point is retrieved when the extractor is removed. The Cancellier extractors can be cleaned with a solvent, e.g. xylene (xylol) and reused.

In a less sophisticated version of this technique, a blunt periodontal irrigating needle or an appropriate size Endo-Eze tip (Ultradent Products Inc., South Jordan, UT, USA) (Fig 6-23) may be used as a substitute for a Cancellier extractor, together with the cyanoacrylate glue. There is no danger of accidental bonding to tooth tissue with this adhesive technique so practitioners should not worry. The worst that can happen is that the silver point resists removal.

Sectional Silver Points

Sectional silver points (Fig 6-24) are very difficult to remove. Provided there is good lighting, visibility and access, removal may be attempted. The approach is still to gain access and loosen the silver point. Specially designed, long reach tips (SybronEndo, Orange, CA, USA) (Fig 6-25) allow the application of ultrasound to whatever is encasing the sectional silver point. A trough may also be made around the coronal end to uncover the sectional silver point. Alternatively, a file or a Masserann extractor may be used to engage the sectional silver point and ultrasonic vibrations from a scaler can be transmitted indirectly. The loosened silver point can then

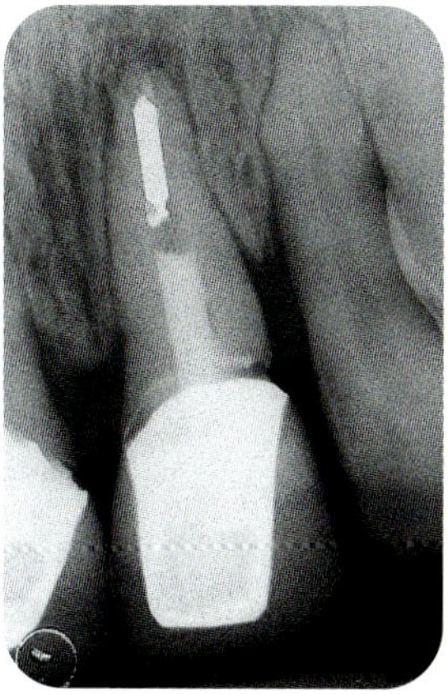

Fig 6-24 Sectional silver point root filling are very difficult to remove.

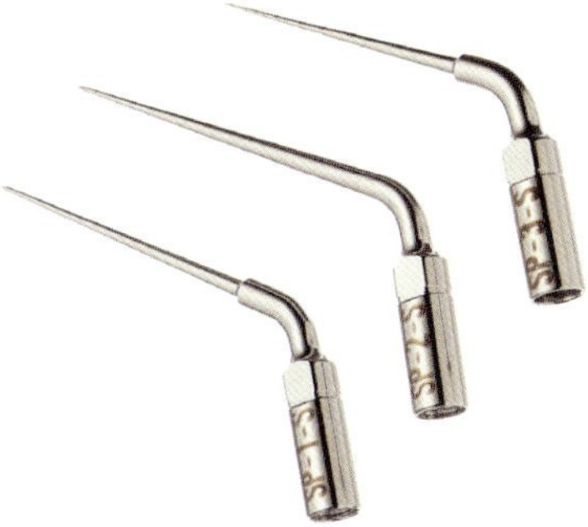

Fig 6-25 Specially designed long reach ultrasonic tips.

be vibrated or floated out using an irrigated ultrasonically activated file. Sometimes, heavily corroded apical sectional silver points will disintegrate when ultrasound is applied.

If an orthograde approach is not successful, then the only option may be to resort to surgery.

Removal of Paste and Cement

The method for the removal of paste or cement root fillings will depend on the type and consistency of the material (Table 6-1):

Soft

The root filling can be removed easily with a hand or rotary file in a similar manner to poorly condensed gutta percha if it is:

- non-setting
- remains soft
- only semi-solid.

Alternatively, it may be washed out, aided by an ultrasonically activated, irrigated file (Fig 6-26).

Table 6-1 **Type of paste/cement root filling material and suggested retreatment technique**

Material	Suggested retreatment technique
Zinc oxide-eugenol cements	May be dissolved with a solvent or removed using ultrasound.
Kri paste	Non-setting, easy to remove with ultrasound.
Zinc phosphate type cement	Not soluble, but will succumb to ultrasound.
SPAD	Bakelite, not soluble, ultrasound helps but removal may be impossible.
AH 26	Non-soluble resin, ultrasound helps but removal may be impossible.
AH Plus	Highly soluble in chloroform.
Endomethasone	Soft, may be removed using a solvent or ultrasound.

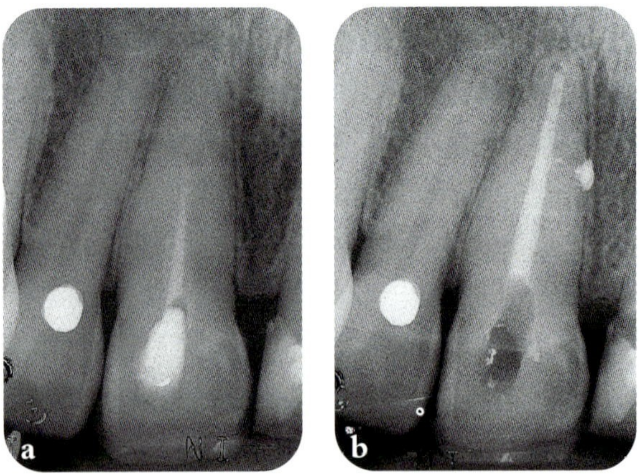

Fig 6-26 Non-surgical retreatment of a paste root filling, removed using ultrasound. (a) Pre-op radiograph. (b) Post-op radiograph.

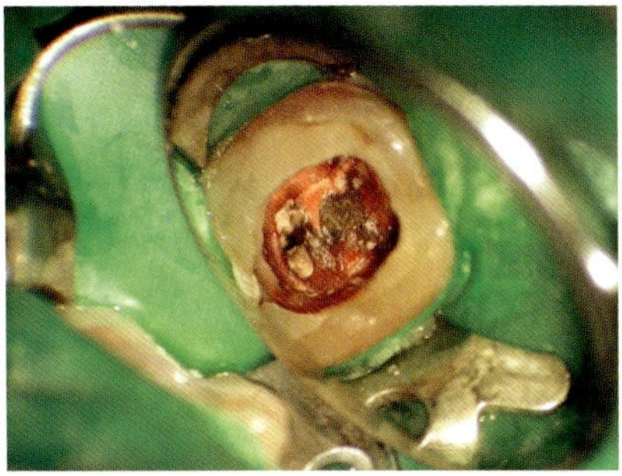

Fig 6-27 Resorcinol-formalin paste root filling when set creates a hard, almost impenetrable barrier and typically staining the tooth a shade of red/pink.

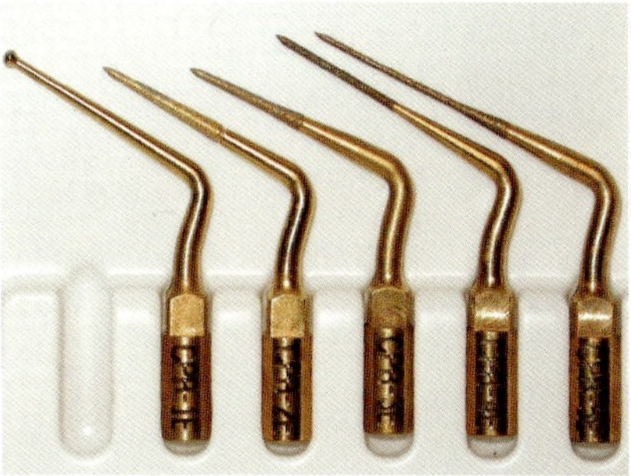

Fig 6-28 Diamond-coated slim ultrasonic tips to aid removal of hard cement root fillings.

Hard

If the paste or cement filling is hard and dense (Fig 6-27), it may need to be removed mechanically by drilling, ultrasonic fragmentation or if soluble, dissolved slowly using an appropriate solvent. The best chance of removing a hard paste or cement root filling is if there are voids present. Drilling with a bur to remove a paste or cement root filling is an extremely hazardous procedure, with the risk of perforation in particular if the canal is curved. Good lighting and magnification are essential adjuncts.

Ultrasonic vibrations can be used to break up paste and cement root fillings and is much safer than drilling with a bur. A powerful piezo-electric machine is especially useful, often combined with special tips which are long, slim and diamond-coated (Fig 6-28). Even when armed with all these tools, removal can still be a slow and laborious process.

Removal of paste and cement root filling with a solvent is also a very slow process and it is often difficult to know which solvent to select for maximum effectiveness. The solvents generally used to dissolve paste and cement root fillings are the same as those for dissolving gutta percha. The technique is similar to that for removal of condensed gutta percha with a solvent. The pulp chamber is first cleared and solvent placed over the root filling. The solvent is worked into the root filling using an endodontic instrument and the softened paste or cement removed gradually. The solvent is replenished as removal progresses.

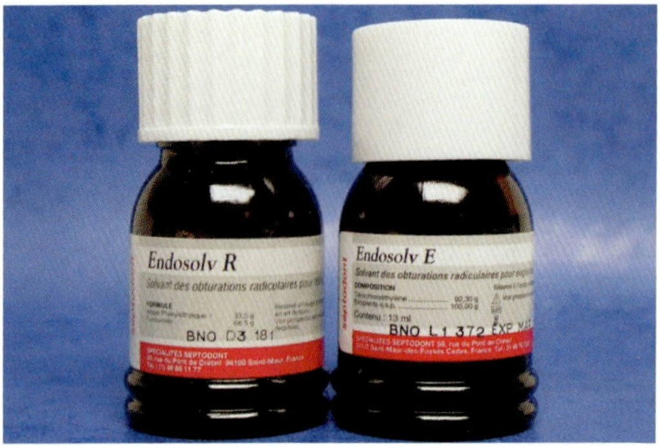

Fig 6-29 Endosolve "R" and "E," commercially available cement/paste solvents.

Endosolv "R" and Endosolv "E" (Spécialités Septodont, Saint-Maur, France) (Fig 6-29) are two solvents formulated specifically for the removal of paste and cement root fillings.

Endosolv "R" is formulated for phenolic resin-type root fillings such as resorcinol-formalin paste (Fig 6-27). Endosolv "E" is formulated for eugenol-based cement root fillings such as Tubli-Seal (Kerr, Orange, CA, USA).

The manufacturers for the solvents have also recommended sealing-in a cotton pellet soaked in the solvent as an interappointment dressing. This is claimed to soften the paste or cement prior to attempted removal, but the speed and depth of penetration is variable.

Unfortunately, not all paste and cement root fillings can be removed. Those that set to give a hard, dense and insoluble root filling may be impossible to remove and surgery may be the only option in such cases.

Conclusions

- The previous root canal filling has to be removed before the root canal system can be negotiated and retreated.
- A variety of methods exists to remove the previous root filling. The choice is dependent on the type of material present.
- Some root filling materials are more difficult to remove than others; some may even defy removal.
- A combination of techniques may be required to achieve a successful result. All techniques require care and patience.

Further Reading

Hülsmann M. The retrieval of silver cones using different techniques. Int Endod J 1990;23:298-303.

Hülsmann M, Stotz S. Efficacy, cleaning ability and safety of different devices for gutta-percha removal in root canal retreatment. Int Endod J 1997;30:227-233.

Vranas RN, Hartwell GR, Moon PC. The effect of endodontic solutions on resorcinol-formalin paste. J Endod 2003;29:69-72.

Wennberg A, Ørstavik D. Evaluation of alternatives to chloroform in endodontic practice. Endod Dent Traumatol 1989;5:234-237.

Wourms DJ, Campbell D, Hicks ML, Pelleu GB. Alternative solvents to chloroform for gutta-percha. J Endod 1990;16:224-226.

Chapter 7

Managing Canal Obstructions

Aim

To describe techniques for managing canal obstructions including broken instruments, blockages and ledges.

Outcome

At the end of this chapter, the practitioner should be aware of techniques to tackle broken instruments, and to overcome blockages and ledges. Effective management of canal obstructions will help secure successful canal negotiation, debridement and retreatment.

Introduction

Sometimes the full length of the root canal system may be inaccessible owing to an obstruction. This may be due to:

- a retained instrument (Fig 7-1)
- blockage of natural tooth substance or foreign material
- a ledge created iatrogenically.

Obstructions may have hindered earlier efforts to achieve infection control and may be a primary factor in causing treatment failure.

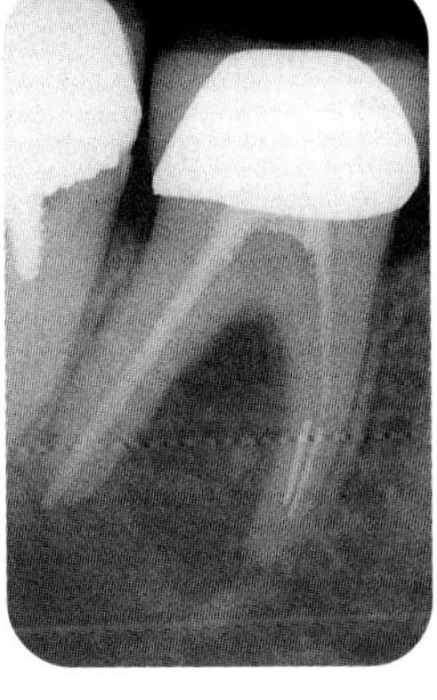

Fig 7-1 Fractured instruments obstructing mesial canals.

General Guidelines

Prevention is better than cure, but canal obstructions can occur despite care and attention. Helpful guidelines to overcome canal obstructions include:

- Acquiring good-quality, angled radiographs to help disclose root curvatures, the location of the blockage and whether the canal is patent below the obstruction.
- Being aware that root canals may be more curved than anticipated. It is important to be aware that canals may have curvatures not only in a mesiodistal but also a buccolingual direction. Think three-dimensionally and try to visualise the root canal morphology.
- Using magnification and additional lighting - being able to see clearly is invaluable when managing obstructions.
- Removing all caries, unsupported tooth structure and restorative materials around the access cavity opening. Clear the pulp chamber of all materials and debris which may fall into the canals by flushing with copious amounts of irrigant; repeat as often as necessary. An ultrasonic scaler is particularly effective for this purpose.
- Widening the coronal access by flaring the canal entrance to allow better visibility and access.
- Improving the radicular access to the level of the obstruction by opening up the glide path as wide as possible for unimpeded straight-line access. This may be carried out using Gates-Glidden burs or NiTi coronal flaring rotary instruments.

Managing Retained Instruments

Ideally, all retained instruments should be removed. However, the management of a retained instrument is very much dependent on its:

- location
- configuration
- material of manufacture.

For example, Hedstrom files are like woodscrews (Fig 7-2) and tend to be very retentive if broken and engaged in dentine. Spiral fillers may act like a spring (Fig 7-3); pulling at the coronal end will merely stretch but not dislodge the instrument. NiTi instruments, being more flexible than those made of stainless steel, are more liable to break off further when inappropriate removal is attempted.

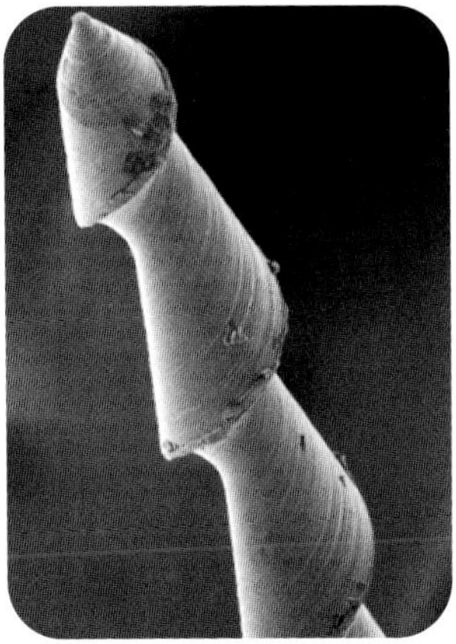

Fig 7-2 Hedstrom files are like woodscrews (SEM).

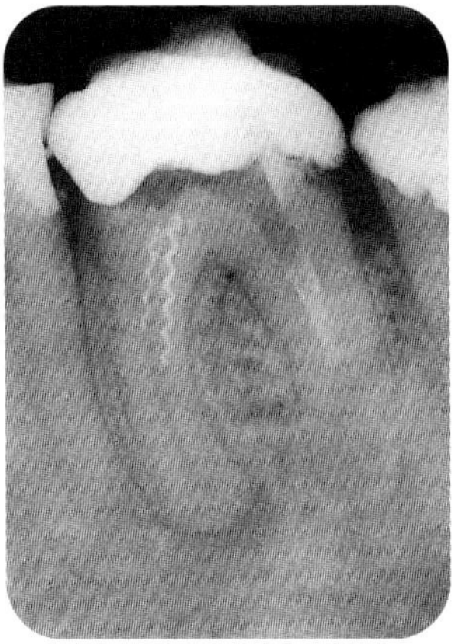

Fig 7-3 Fractured spiral fillers obstructing mesial canals.

The consequences of leaving a retained instrument is critically dependent on the microbial status of the canal when the procedural accident occurred. The microbial status is dependent on the:

- pretreatment pulpal state
- presence or absence of a periapical radiolucency.

In general, if instrument separation occurs during the treatment of a vital pulp, provided the root canal system is not opened to microbial ingress, the long-term prognosis remains good. On the other hand, in cases of established apical periodontitis, retrieval of a broken instrument is highly desirable, if not essential, for a predictable biological outcome (Fig 7-4). Relying on the separated instrument to provide an effective apical seal is often fanciful and infection is likely to persist. Surgery may be the only option if an instrument is protruding beyond the apical foramen and not amenable to retrieval by non-surgical means (Fig 7-5). General guidelines for management of canals obstructed by foreign objects are set out in Table 7-1.

If Retrievable

Initially, attempts should be made to retrieve the retained instrument from the root canal – in particular, if it is in the coronal part of the canal. Most of the techniques and devices applicable have been covered in Chapter 6. The procedure consists of three stages.

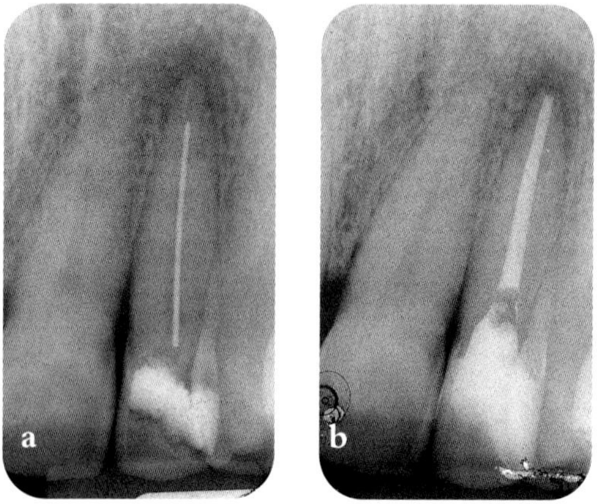

Fig 7-4 Fractured instrument in a tooth with apical periodontitis should be retrieved and retreated as it cannot provide a reliable and effective apical seal. (a) Pre-op radiograph. (b) Post-op radiograph.

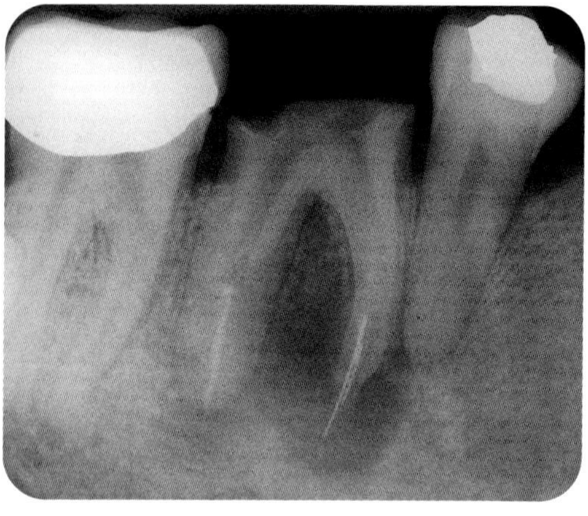

Fig 7-5 Surgery may be the only option if fractured instruments are protruding into the periapex.

Stage 1: Expose the coronal end

A "staging platform" is made (Fig 7-6a, b) at the coronal end of the retained instrument, with a Gates-Glidden "belly" bur (Fig 7-7), modified by flattening off its guiding tip. NiTi coronal flaring rotary instruments may also be similarly modified and used.

Dentine around the top of the retained instrument is carefully removed, creating a trough. This may be achieved using:

- a small round bur
- a Meitrac or Masserann trepan
- ultrasound, preferably (Fig 7-6c).

Table 7-1 **Guidelines for the management of canals obstructed by foreign objects**

Level of obstruction	Procedure
Coronal part of canal	
All cases	Retrieval followed by retreatment.
Middle third of canal	
Possible to retrieve	Retrieval followed by retreatment.
Impossible to retrieve, but can bypass	Bypass, retreat and incorporate into the root filling.
Impossible to bypass	Retreat to level of obstruction and review. Surgical retreatment may be indicated subsequently.
Apical third of canal	
Possible to retrieve	Retrieval followed by retreatment.
Impossible to retrieve, but can bypass	Bypass, retreat and incorporate into the root filling.
Impossible to bypass, tight seal by object	Retreat to level of obstruction and review.
Impossible to bypass, lack of effective seal	Retreat to level of obstruction and review, follow-up surgery if indicated.
Object protruding through apical foramen	Retreat to level of obstruction followed by surgery if then indicated.

Stage 2: Loosen the instrument

The instrument lodged in the root canal must first be loosened. This may be achieved with small hand or rotary files and a gel-form chelating agent to lubricate the file and soften the dentine. If the obstruction is a small fragment of an instrument, ultrasonic or sonic vibrations may be used to try and loosen and eventually float it out.

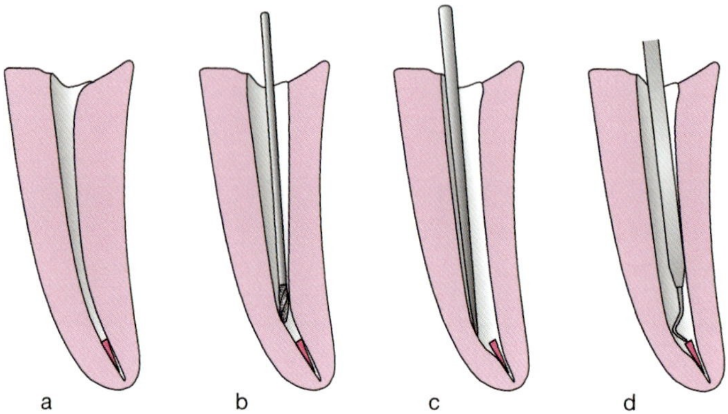

Fig 7-6 Retrieval of a fractured instrument. (a) An instrument fragment in apical third of the root canal. (b) A Gates-Glidden belly bur is used to create a "staging platform". (c) Ultrasound is used to create a trough and loosen the instrument. (d) A Cancellier is used to extract the instrument.

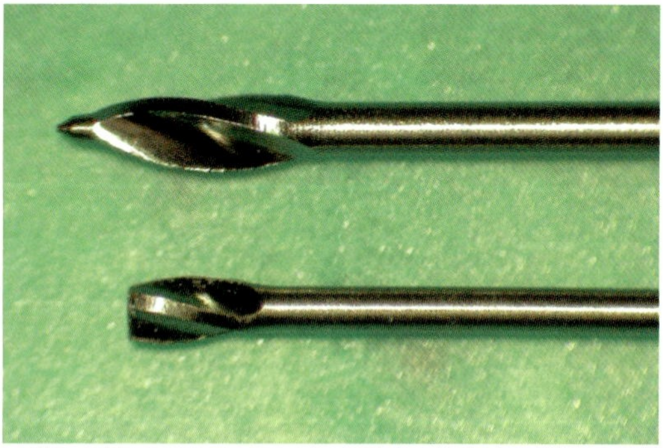

Fig 7-7 Gates-Glidden bur (top) and modified belly bur (bottom).

Stage 3: Engage the instrument

Once a sufficient length of the instrument has been uncovered, it can then be engaged and removed using:

- Hedstrom files
- Steiglitz forceps
- Masserann or Meitrac extractors (see Chapter 6)
- Others devices – Cancellier extractor (See Chapter 6) and Ruddle iRS (instrument removal system).

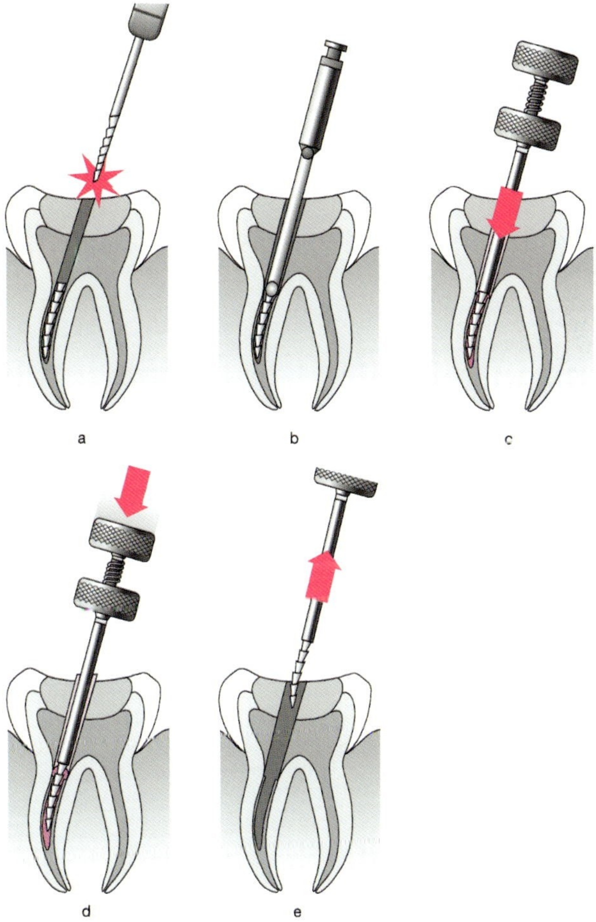

Fig 7-8 Removal of a fractured file instrument using the Meitrac system. (a) File fractured. (b) Trephining bur to remove dentine and uncover the coronal end of the file. (c) Extractor of appropriate size is placed over the exposed end. (d) Top of the extractor is pressed down and rotated gently to engage the top of the file. (e) Both sections of the extractor are squeezed together and the file withdrawn when the extractor is removed.

The procedure for the removal of a retained instrument using the Meitrac system is shown in Fig 7-8. If the separated instrument is loose but not free, a Cancellier extractor (Fig 7-6d) may be used.

The Ruddle iRS (Dentsply Maillefer, Ballaigues, Switzerland) is another extractor device. It consists of a hollow tube with a side cut out. The tube is placed over the fragment of instrument. A stylet is then inserted into the hollow tube to engage the instrument, which is removed when the assembly is withdrawn.

Unfortunately, there are frustrating practical limits to these methods of instrument removal. For example, even the finest-beaked Steiglitz forceps are often unable to reach deep enough to grasp a retained instrument, or an inadequate length of instrument can be exposed or available coronally to allow secure engagement of a Masserann or Meitrac extractor.

If Not Retrievable

If retrieval is impossible or too risky, the next best scenario is to bypass (Fig 7-9) and incorporate the retained instrument into the new root filling. Stainless steel and NiTi instruments will not corrode if left inside a root canal. They are, therefore, relatively harmless in themselves; it is the infected canal apical to the obstruction that is the problem. The technique for bypassing a retained instrument is the same as that for managing a blockage or ledge.

If it is impossible to retrieve or bypass, then there is no alternative but to leave the broken instrument inside the root canal and retreat the tooth to the level of the obstruction. Sometimes, it may be possible for irrigants and medicaments to penetrate past the broken instrument so the canal should be soaked with copious amounts of sodium hypochlorite and dressed to help reduce the intracanal microbial load before inserting the root filling. After completion of non-surgical retreatment, the tooth

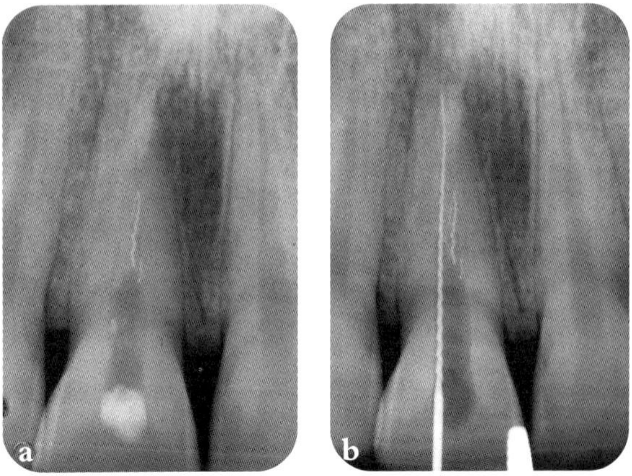

Fig 7-9 Bypassing a fractured file. (a) The file fragment lodged in the wall of the root canal. (b) The obstruction bypassed and the canal negotiated.

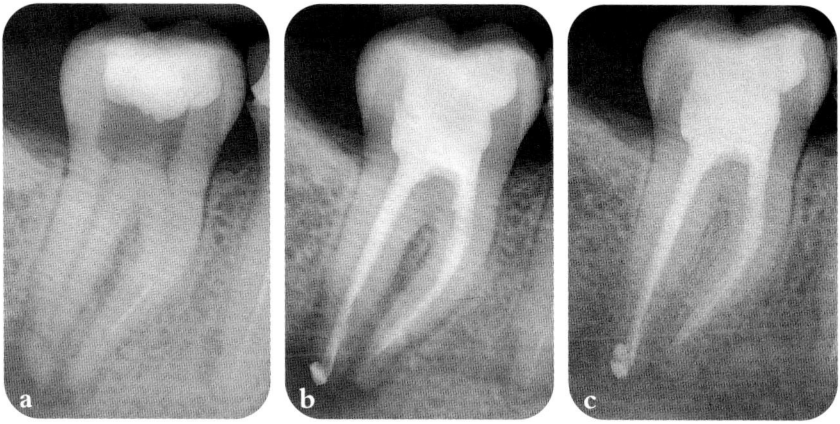

Fig 7-10 A retained instrument may not necessarily jeopardise the success of non-surgical retreatment. (a) A broken fragment of instrument lodged in a mesial canal. (b) Instrument bypassed and incorporated into root filling. (c) Review two years later.

should be restored with a long-term temporary restoration and put on probation, for up to a year initially, to see if the symptoms resolve and healing occurs (see Chapter 1, ESE guidelines). If not, follow-up treatment, possibly surgery, may be required. With careful case selection (see Chapter 3) the success rate of retreatment of teeth with retained instruments may not be significantly reduced (Fig 7-10).

Managing Blockages and Ledges

A blockage is an obstruction in a previously patent canal, preventing an instrument from reaching the apex. It may be due to compaction of:

- dentinal debris
- restorative material
- root filling material
- foreign bodies (e.g. cotton wool).

A ledge is an artificially created canal irregularity, altering the natural canal path, obstructing access to the apex in an otherwise patent canal. Ledging results from a combination of:

- selecting an excessively large and inflexible instrument for the curvature of the canal
- use of instruments with sharp, cutting tips
- not precurving or overcurving instruments

- the use of excessive apical force
- inappropriate-directed clockwise rotations as opposed to safer, controlled, balanced force rotations.

The procedure to tackle a blockage or ledge is as follows:

Instrument Selection

- Hand instruments provide better tactile feedback and are preferable to rotary instruments for overcoming a blockage or ledge.
- The shortest instrument that can reach the level of the blockage or ledge but not necessarily the apex should be chosen. Shorter instruments are stiffer and less likely to buckle. Longer instruments that will reach the apex are only required after the blockage or ledge is overcome.
- Larger size instruments are stiffer but are less manoeuvrable within the tight confines of a canal, and may be too wide to pass to the level of the obstruction.
- The type of hand instrument, design and material from which it is manufactured, have bearings on its suitability. NiTi files are not so easy to precurve. K-type files are stiffer and more robust than Hedstrom files. Carbon steel instruments are stiffer than stainless steel instruments which, in turn, are stiffer than those made of NiTi. Specially manufactured "pathfinding" files (e.g. Pathfinder-CS, Kerr, Orange, CA, USA; C+ file, Dentsply Maillefer, Ballaigues, Switzerland) (Fig 7-11), which are more resistant to buckling, are available and helpful.
- Ultrasonic instrumentation has been advocated for managing blockages. The biophysical effects of cavitation and acoustic microstreaming generated by ultrasound may help dislodge the obstruction. Ultrasonic instruments are not necessarily superior to hand instruments.

Technique

- Before the instrument is inserted into the root canal, it should be precurved to the extent of the expected curvature of the canal. Occasionally, an acute curve (Fig 7-12) placed in the last 3–4 mm of the instrument may be helpful (Fig 7-13). Many files are fitted with directional stops to aid correct orientation of the precurved file.
- The instrument should be used like a "pick" in a "watch-winding" motion (Fig 7-14). The instrument is twiddled between the finger and thumb, and advanced with minimal vertical pressure. The instrument is "walked" in a clockwise direction when advanced to detect when it "catches" the obstruction. When the instrument binds, pull back slightly, freeing the instrument and advance again in short "pecking" action. The aim is to try and slide the

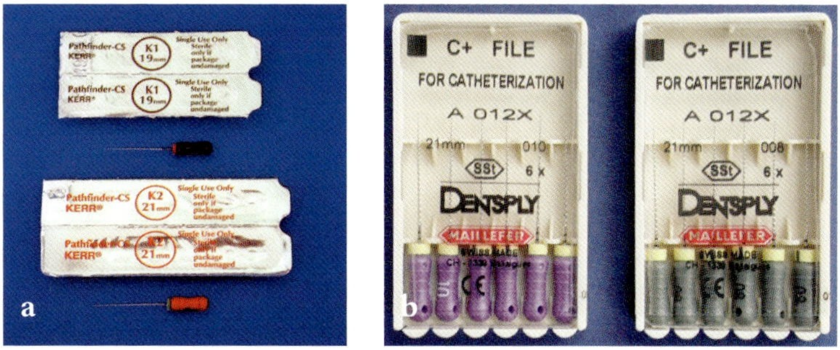

Fig 7-11 Specially manufactured files to help canal negotiation. (a) Pathfinder-CS files. (b) C+ files.

Fig 7-12 Small file with an acute curve to help negotiate a ledged canal.

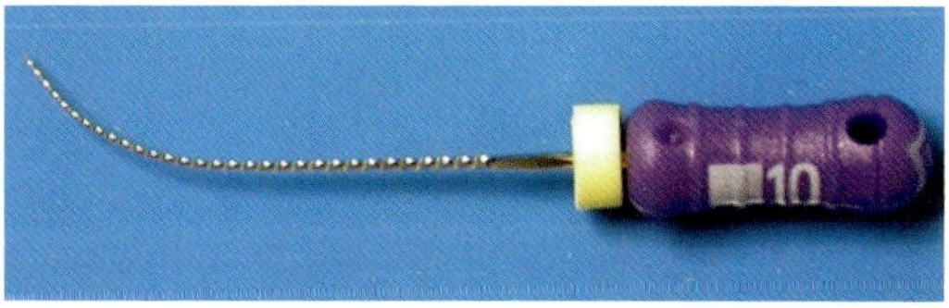

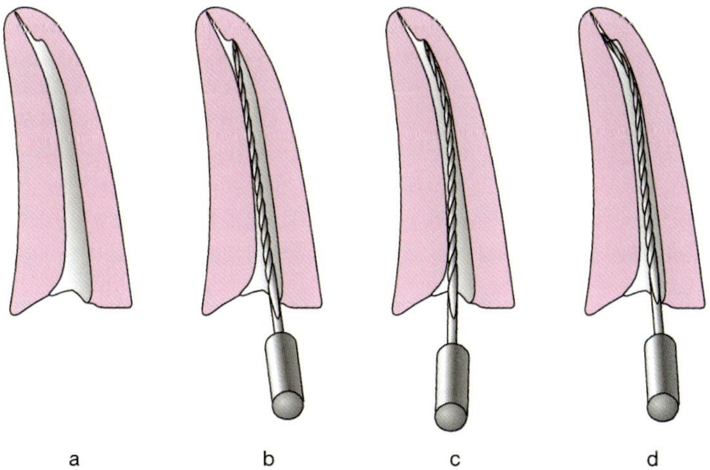

Fig 7-13 Overcoming a ledge. (a) Ledged canal. (b) A straight instrument is unable to negotiate the ledge. (c) A gently curved instrument may be equally unsuccessful. (d) With a more acute curve, the instrument may be able to negotiate past the ledge.

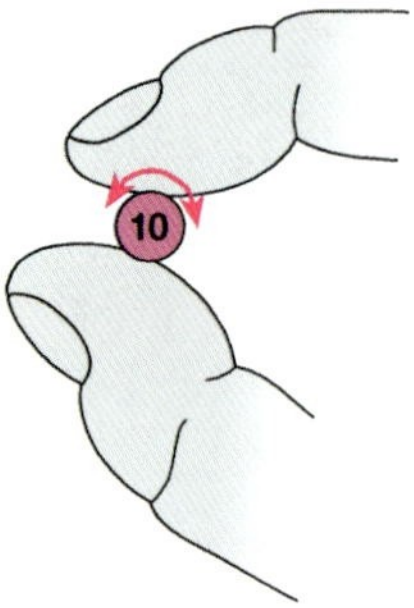

Fig 7-14 Watch-winding an instrument to overcome an intracanal obstruction.

instrument past the blockage or ledge gradually. The instrument should not be rotated excessively to avoid instrument separation. When the instrument is withdrawn, it should be inspected carefully for signs of "wind-up" or "unwinding" (Fig 7-15) indicating a risk of imminent fracture.

- Chelating agents soften dentine and lubricate the canal but are only useful when the instrument is making apical progress, past the blockage or ledge. Then a small amount of chelating agent, preferably in a viscous gel-form, may be introduced into the canal. It is pointless to flood the root canals with chelating agent in the futile hope that it will "dissolve" the obstruction.
- Once the blockage or ledge is overcome, the patent canal should be instrumented with care, slowly, in short circumferential filing strokes, to rasp away the ledge and open up the canal progressively.
- If all obstructions have been overcome, the canal can now be cleaned, shaped and filled by conventional means (Fig 7-16).
- If an instrument cannot overcome a blockage or ledge, it may still be possible for irrigants and medicaments to penetrate past the obstruc-

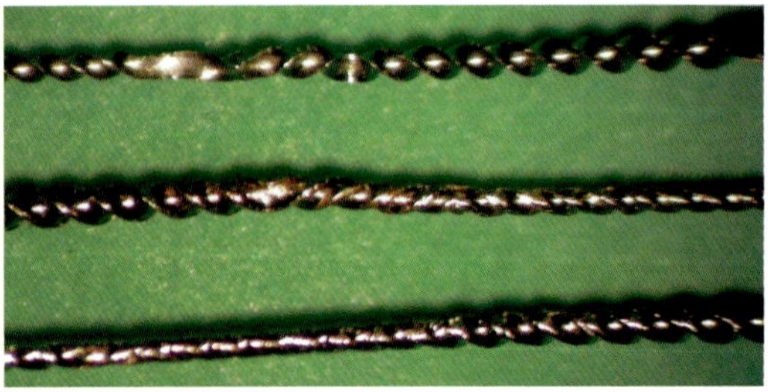

Fig 7-15 Instruments showing signs of "wind-up" or "unwinding", indicating the risk of imminent file fracture.

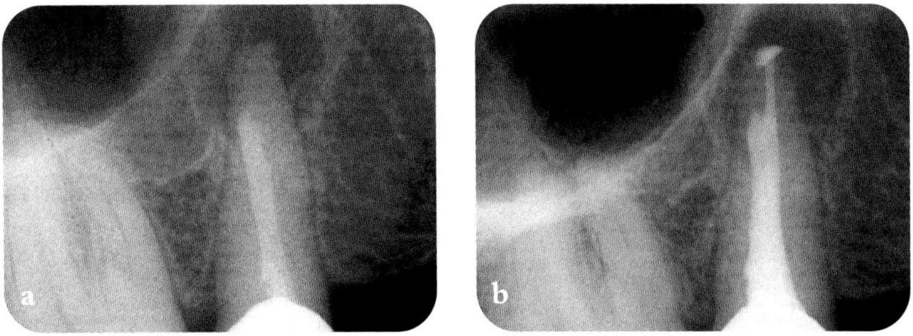

Fig 7-16 Successful non-surgical retreatment of a ledged canal. (a) Pre-op radiograph. (b) Post-op radiograph.

tion. The canal to the level of the obstruction should therefore be soaked with generous amounts of sodium hypochlorite and, if considered appropriate, dressed for an extended period to maximise disinfection.

- The canal should then be obturated to the level of the obstruction (Fig 7-17). Warm gutta percha techniques provide the best three-dimensional seal. In wide canals or in cases in which apical damage has occurred (see Chapter 4,

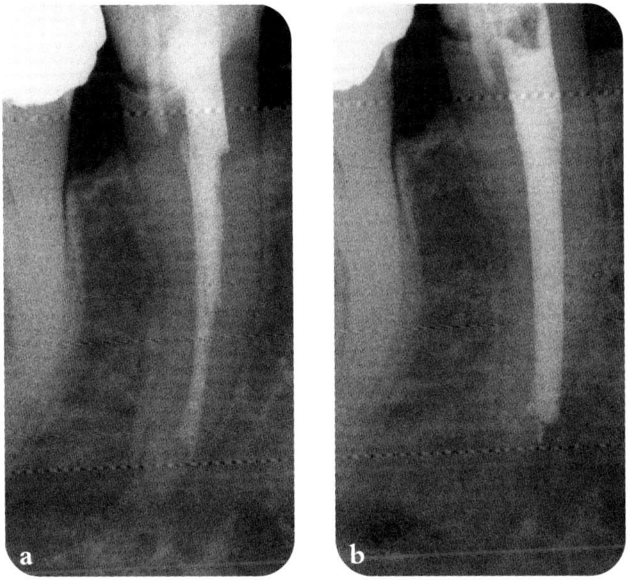

Fig 7-17 Canal obturated to level of obstruction if it cannot be overcome. (a) Pre-op radiograph. (b) Post-op radiograph.

Fig 4-7), or if immediate follow-up surgery is planned, the canal may be filled with MTA (see Chapter 8) instead of gutta percha.
- Afterwards, the tooth should be restored with a long-term temporary restoration and monitored, initially for up to a year. Any follow-up treatment that may be required will be dependent on any sign or symptoms; surgery or extraction may be needed.

Conclusions

- Canal obstructions due to broken instruments, blockages and ledges are usually a result of procedural errors.
- A retained instrument should be removed but if this is not possible the next best scenario is to bypass and incorporate the instrument in the root filling.
- If an obstruction cannot be overcome or bypassed, then the canal should be thoroughly cleaned and well-obturated to the level of the obstruction. The tooth should then be monitored.
- Surgery or, at worst, extraction may be necessary if an obstructed canal cannot be managed successfully and gives rise to symptoms.

Further Reading

Åkerblom A, Hasselgren G. The prognosis of endodontic treatment of obliterated root canals. J Endod 1988;14:565-567.

Fors UGH, Berg J.-O. Endodontic treatment of root canals obstructed by foreign objects. Int Endod J 1986;19:2-10.

Grossman LI. Fate of endodontically treated teeth with fractured root canal instruments. J Brit Endod Soc 1969;2:35-37.

Ruddle CJ. Broken instrument removal: The endodontic challenge. Dentistry Today 2002;21:70-81

Chapter 8

A Surgical Alternative

Aim

To outline the rationale and describe step-by-step the apicectomy and root-end filling procedure.

Outcome

At the end of this chapter, the practitioner should be familiar with the planning process, preparatory measures and the practical procedure of apicectomy and root-end filling in managing endodontic failure.

Introduction

Surgical retreatment encompasses a number of procedures, referred to synonymously as:

- periapical curettage/periradicular curettage
- apicectomy/root end resection/apical resection
- root-end filling/retrograde filling
- surgical repair
- root resection/root amputation
- hemisection/bicuspidization.

As it is beyond the remit of this book to cover all these procedures, the focus of this chapter will be on apicectomy and root-end filling - the most frequently performed endodontic surgical retreatment procedure. In this chapter, reference to surgery should be taken to mean apicectomy and root-end filling.

Apicectomy and Root-End Filling

Rationale

As far as endodontic failures are concerned, an apicectomy is indicated:

- when conventional orthograde root canal treatment or non-surgical retreatment is impractical (Fig 8-1)

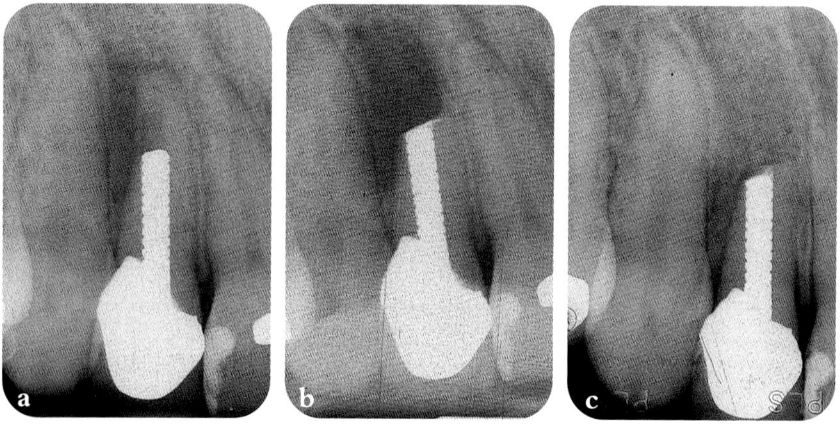

Fig 8-1 Surgery indicated when non-surgical retreatment impracticable. (a) Tooth with large threaded post. (b) Apicectomy performed and MTA root-end filling placed. (b) One-year review.

- following the failure of conventional root canal treatment or non-surgical retreatment (Fig 8-2)
- as an adjunct to non-surgical retreatment, e.g., to correct procedural errors (Fig 8-3)
- when biopsy or exploratory investigation is indicated, e.g., to manage a cyst or other suspect lesions (Fig 8-4).

Apicectomy is primarily designed to remove the portion of root apex that is inaccessible to instrumentation and, as a consequence, cannot be cleaned, shaped or filled, or is associated with extraradicular infection (Fig 8-5), which is unresponsive to conventional orthograde treatment. During apicectomy, any overextended root filling and pathological tissues may be removed. A root-end filling is then placed to create a seal at the cut root end. The intention is to eliminate microorganisms in the untreated apical few millimetres, or imprison and seal them within the root canal system preventing their leakage. Deprived of sustenance and unable to cause any harmful effects, most microorganisms may eventually die. Unfortunately, it is now realised that such a premise is flawed because unless the root canal is properly cleaned, shaped and filled, even after apicectomy and placement of a root-end filling, viable microorganisms may still persist within the root canal system and cause apical periodontitis (Fig 8-6). Even if the root canal is not negotiable to the apex, a good-quality root filling should still be placed as far down as possible prior to surgery. This is considered crucial to a successful surgical outcome. Good surgical skill alone is insufficient to ensure success; correct case selection, thorough examination and an

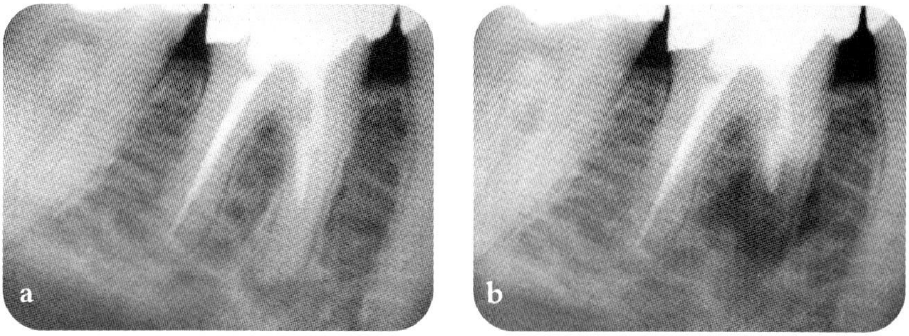

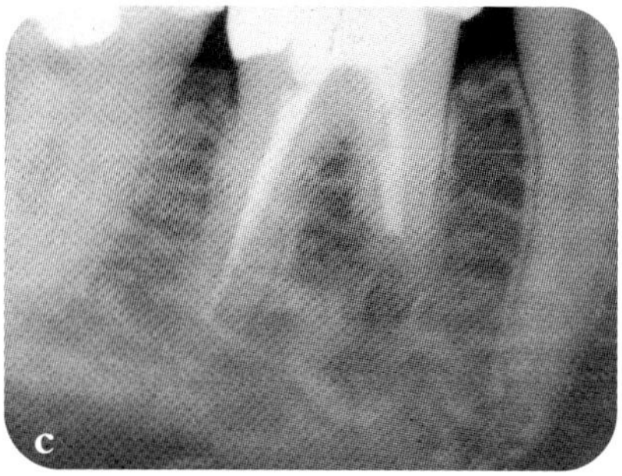

Fig 8-2 Surgery following unsuccessful non-surgical retreatment. (a) Mesial canals not completely negotiable. (b) Mesial root apicected to level of orthograde root filling, no root-end filling necessary. (c) Six-month review.

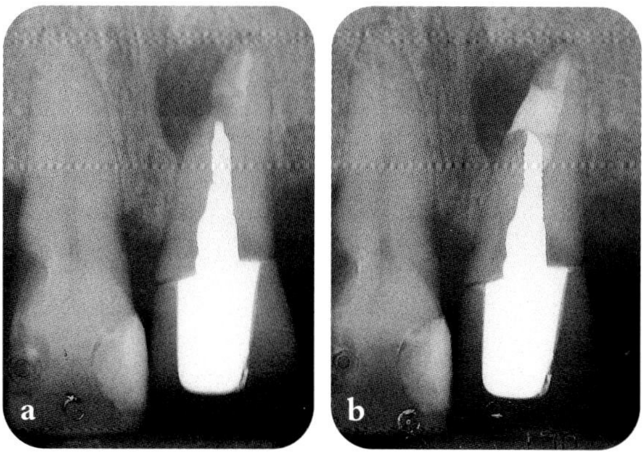

Fig 8-3 Correction of procedural error. (a) Post space perforation. (b) Postsurgical repair.

understanding of the biological basis of treatment are important. On the other hand, the presence of a complex coronal restoration or post can no longer be regarded as justification for the surgical approach, which is now rarely the recommended first line of management in endodontic failure. Readers may like to refer to Chapter 3 on the relative merits and limitations of surgery.

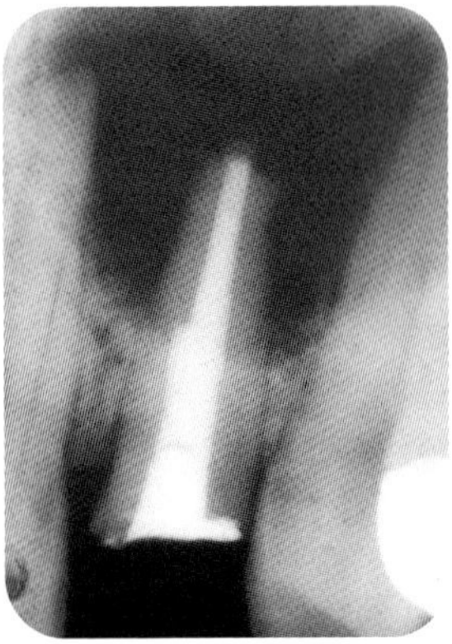

Fig 8-4 Surgery indicated for biopsy and exploration of a large periapical lesion.

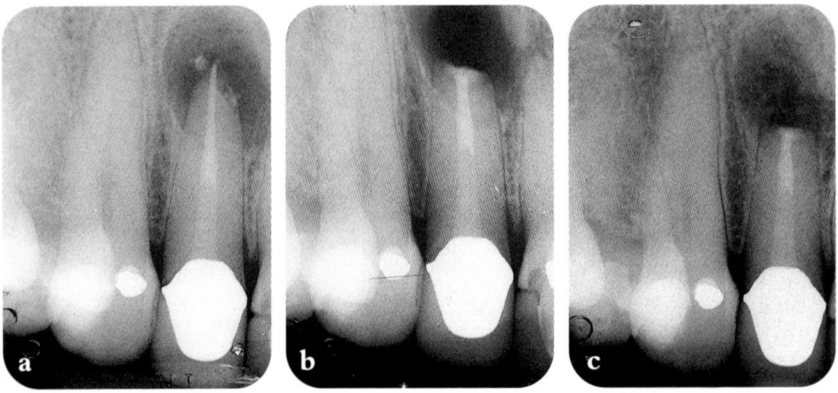

Fig 8-5 Surgical management of suspected extraradicular infection. (a) An overextended root filling and a periapical lesion. (b) Apicectomy, periapical curettage and root-end filling performed. Biopsy report confirmed extraradicular infection caused by actinomyces. (c) Review six months later.

Medical and Dental Considerations

Medical and dental considerations are included as part of the preoperative assessment, as for any surgical procedure. The patient's physician should be consulted if appropriate. The relevant radiographs should have been taken, possible complications clarified, prognosis explained and informed consent obtained.

General considerations for endodontic surgery are similar to those for tooth extraction.

Local considerations include the following:

- access and visibility including sulcus depth

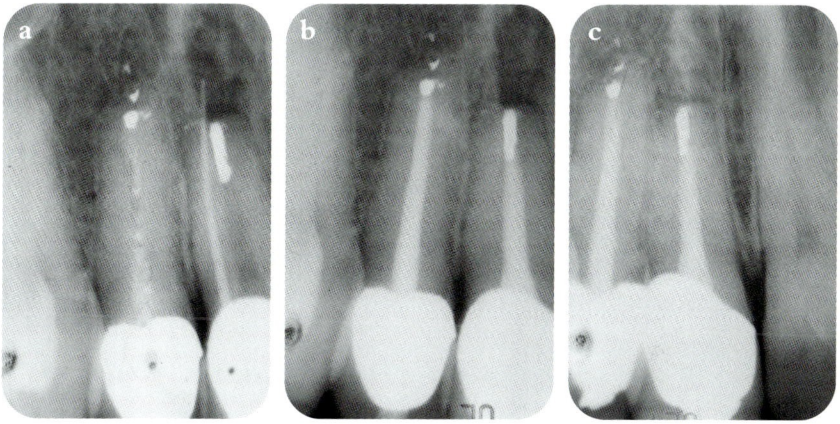

Fig 8-6 Apicectomy and root-end filling will not eliminate the reservoir of infection within the root canal system. (a) Failure following surgery, a gutta percha cone in the sinus tract. (b) Following non-surgical retreatment. (c) Review one year later.

- location and proximity of neurovascular bundles
- anatomical structures including fraenal and muscle attachments
- quality and quantity of periodontal support.

Preoperative Preparations

- Patients should be advised to dress comfortably and, if necessary, an escort should be arranged to take them home afterwards.
- Practise pre-emptive analgesia. Analgesics are more effective if taken prior to anticipated pain. So, if able to tolerate non-steroidal anti-inflammatory drugs (NSAID), the patient should take Ibuprofen 400 mg one hour before their appointment.
- To reduce the risk of infection, the patient should be given an antiseptic mouthwash of chlorhexidine gluconate 0.2% (Corsodyl, GlaxoSmithKline, Brentford, Middlesex, UK) (Fig 8-7) to rinse for 1 min, before the commencement of surgery. Sometimes, the patient may be instructed to start the chlorhexidine mouthwash two days before surgery to reduce the oral flora and plaque formation.

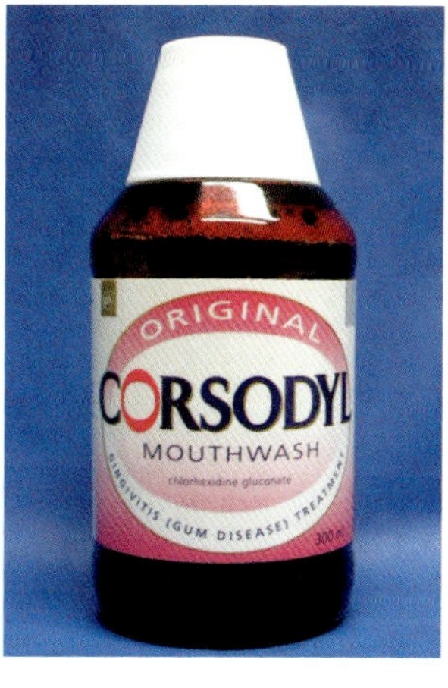

Fig 8-7 Chlorhexidine antiseptic mouthwash.

Surgical Kit

A basic surgical kit should be assembled; individual practitioners will have preferences for particular instruments. An example of a surgical set-up containing instruments mentioned in this chapter is shown in Fig 8-8.

Anaesthesia

Surgery is normally performed under local anaesthesia, but in the case of very anxious patients, conscious sedation may be arranged. General anaesthesia is seldom indicated and is preferably avoided since there is better control of the surgical field under local anaesthesia.

In general, the local anaesthesia required for apicectomy and root-end filling is the same as for tooth extraction. In the mandible, regional block anaesthesia must be administered and the tissues around the operation area also infiltrated with local anaesthetic solution. In the maxilla, buccal and palatal infiltration anaesthesia is required. In the anterior maxilla, the incisive papilla

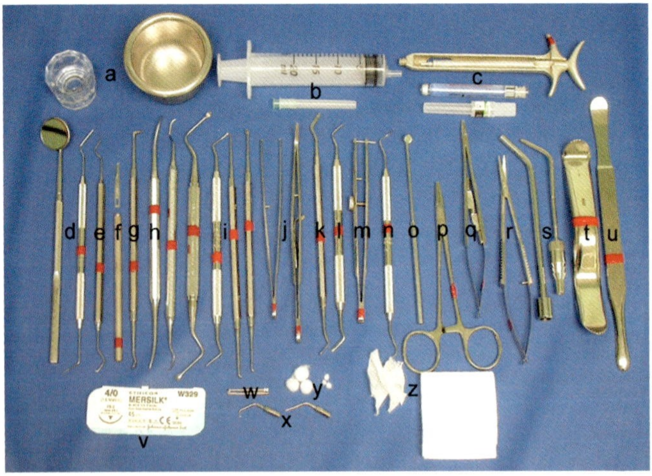

Fig 8-8 Example of surgical set-up. (a) Dappen dish and saline bowl. (b) Irrigating syringe and needle. (c) Local anaesthetic syringe, cartridge and needle. (d) Front surface mirror and DG16 endodontic explorer. (e) Briault probe. (f) Microsurgical blade and handle. (g) Mitchell's trimmer. (h) Molt periosteal elevator. (i) Selection of surgical curettes. (j) Tissue forceps and locking tweezers. (k) Flat plastic. (l) Hollenback carver. (m) Root-end filling carrier. (n) Root-end filling plugger. (o) Micro-mirror. (p) Surgical haemostat. (q) Castroviejo needle holder. (r) Castroviejo scissors. (s) Suction tips. (t) Minnesota retractor. (u) Seldin retractor. (v) Silk suture. (w) Round and fissure surgical burs (Ash TC RA No. 8 round & No. 702 fissure burs). (x) Ultrasonic micro-tips. (y) Cotton pellets. (z) Ribbon gauze and square gauze.

and canal will need to be anaesthetized as well. With infiltration anaesthesia, care should be exercised not to inject into the surrounding skeletal muscle or bleeding may be increased.

Local anaesthetic solutions of 2% lidocaine (lignocaine) with 1:80,000 adrenaline should provide effective anaesthesia and haemostasis. Formulations with 1:50,000 adrenaline (Fig 8-9), if available, are even more effective in controlling haemorrhage. A sufficient amount of local anaesthetic solution, typically 3–5 mL in a healthy individual, must be administered to ensure a bloodless field and profound anaesthesia during the whole procedure. Local anaesthetic solutions containing the synthetic polypeptide vasoconstrictor felypressin (octapressin) do not provide adequate haemostasis and should be avoided if possible.

Flap Design and Reflection

Tissue flaps vary in designs, shapes and sizes. Whichever design is chosen should always fulfil the well-established surgical principles:

- ensuring there is adequate blood supply to permit good healing
- siting the edges of the flap to lie on sound bone to prevent breakdown of the flap margins (Fig 8-10); bony dehiscence and fenestration should be avoided
- avoiding small flaps which will be bruised, stretched and torn in an effort to achieve good surgical access and unobstructed vision
- remembering that flaps heal across the thickness of the wound, not the perimeter; larger, more adequate flaps are preferred
- maintaining the integrity of interdental papillae and avoiding sharp angles

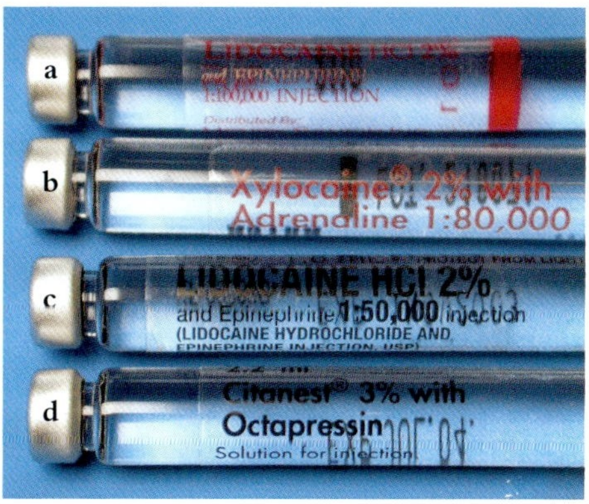

Fig 8-9 Local anaesthetic solutions with (a) 1:100000; (b) 1:80000; or (c) 1:50000 adrenaline and (d) synthetic polypeptide vasoconstrictor felypressin (octapressin).

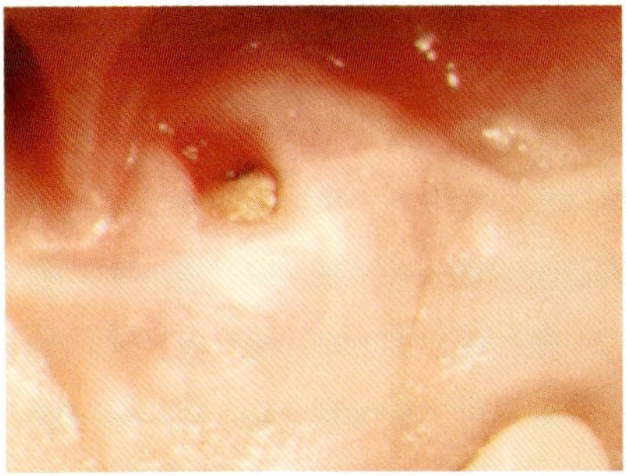

Fig 8-10 Mucosal defect exposing root end as a result of inappropriate flap design and soft tissue management.

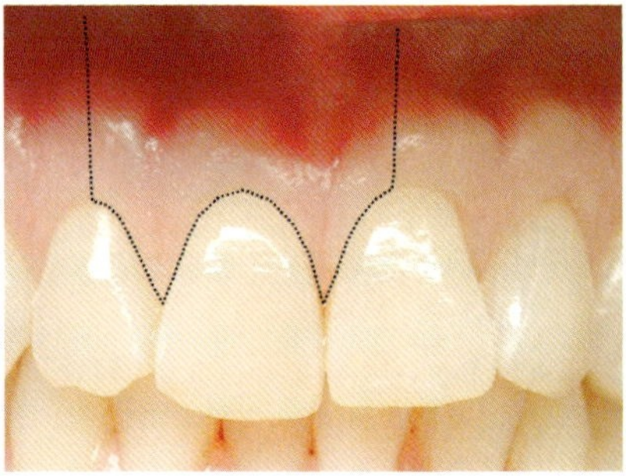

Fig 8-11 Outline of incision for an intrasulcular mucoperiosteal flap.

- placing incisions accurately and cutting through periosteum
- reflecting the flap cleanly and with minimum trauma to the tissues.

An intrasulcular full-thickness mucoperiosteal tissue flap (Fig 8-11) provides excellent access and visibility, with minimal to no scarring and good healing. To facilitate better tissue approximation which enhances healing, the incision lines should be made with a single, firm cut with a scalpel. Microsurgical scalpels (Swann-Morton Ltd., Sheffield, UK) (Fig 8-12) are available in different shapes, some double-edged. These smaller blades make it easier getting into the interproximal spaces and are also excellent for ensuring that the incisions follow the irregular contours of the underlying bone without slipping. The number of relieving incisions is dependent on the surgical access required. The relieving incisions should be made first, extending into the gingival crevice and including the gingival papilla. Relieving incisions should be vertical, not angled, as this will limit the number of vertically-running blood vessels severed, reducing the potential for haemorrhage. The horizontal incision is then made along the gingival crevice to join the vertical relieving incisions.

A Mitchell's trimmer is used to reflect the tissue flap by lifting the periosteum from the bone at a vertical incision line (Fig 8-13). By slowly undermining the flap in a coronal direction, easing the periosteum off bone, the whole tissue flap is gently reflected. The flap should not be reflected from the gingival papilla or anywhere along the horizontal incision. Most periosteal elevators are too large and their use will crush, tear and damage the delicate gingival tissues, particularly the papillae. Once reflected, the flap should be protected with tissue retrac-

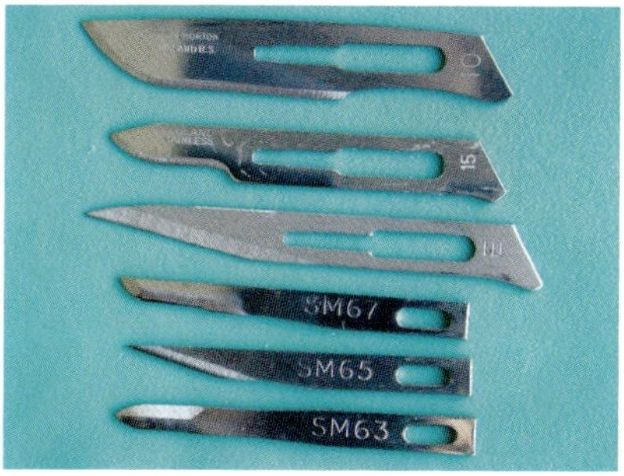

Fig 8-12 Microsurgical scalpel blades (bottom three) are smaller than conventional, normal size blades (top three).

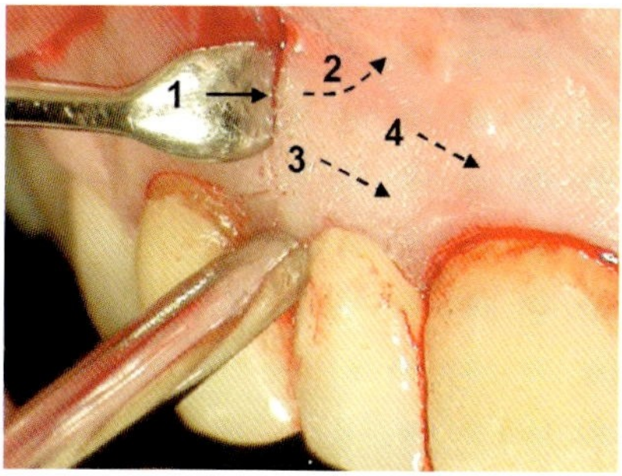

Fig 8-13 Sequence of flap reflection. Begin at the middle of the vertical relieving incision (1), the flap is undermined (2) and elevated (3,4).

tors. For improved access and visibility, and to prevent excessive pulling of the tissue flap, surgery on anterior teeth may be performed with the patient's mouth closed, biting on a piece of gauze.

In cases in which crowns are present, a particular concern may be to preserve the aesthetics by avoiding flaps involving the marginal gingiva and interdental papilla. One such design, the submarginal rectangular flap, also referred to as the Luebke-Ochsenbein (Fig 8-14), consists of a scalloped, horizontal incision in the attached gingiva, following the marginal gingiva contour, with two vertical relieving incisions. An adequate width of attached gingiva, preferably 5 mm, is needed to prevent ischaemia of the remaining attached gingiva. Also, the surgical bony access must not extend to the incision line and the submarginal rectangular flap design is recommended in the maxilla only. Another disadvantage is that there is a greater tendency to scarring. A "papilla base incision" (Fig 8-15) has also been advocated to avoid and preserve the interdental papilla.

Locating the Tooth Apex

The periapical lesion may have perforated the buccal cortical plate making location of the apex simple. However, if the apex is still covered by thick cortical bone then bone removal is necessary. The advent of implants has resulted in the availability of many surgical handpieces (Fig 8-16); their torque and speed control features plus effective coolant delivery make them perfect for apicectomies. High-speed air-driven turbines are also available (e.g. Impact Air 45, Palisades Dental, Tenafly, NJ, USA) (Fig 8-17) in which the head of the handpiece is orientated at a 45° angle to improve access, a

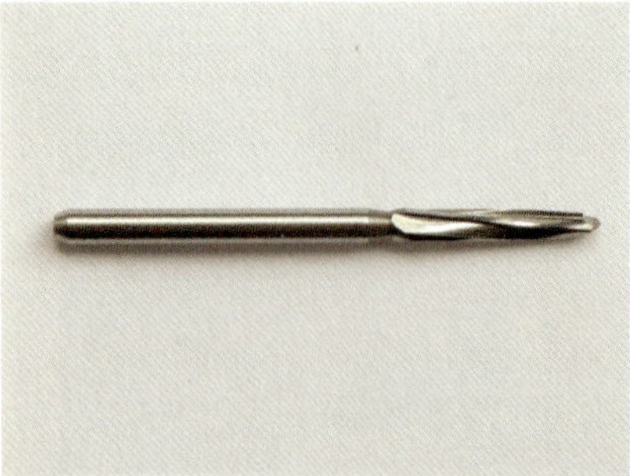

Fig 8-19 Lindemann bone cutting bur.

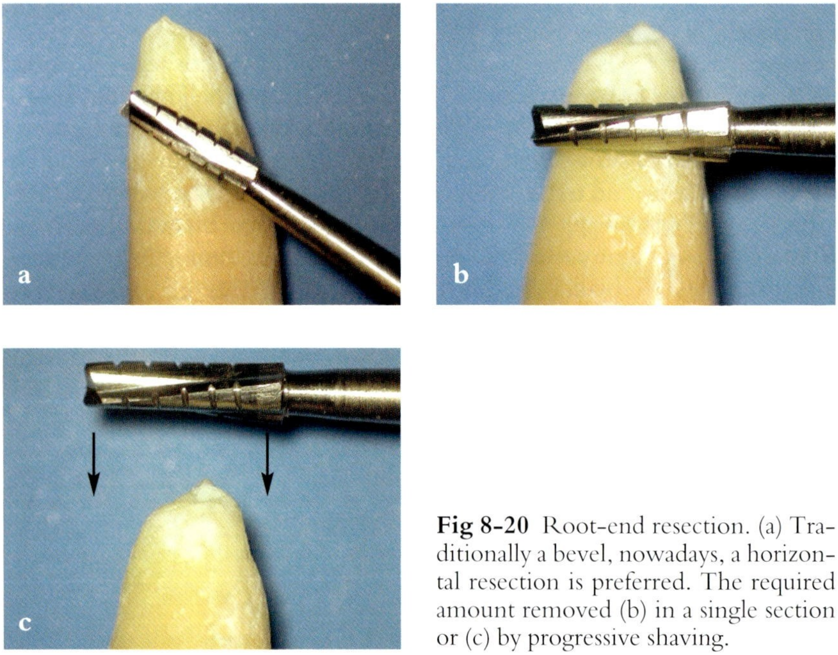

Fig 8-20 Root-end resection. (a) Traditionally a bevel, nowadays, a horizontal resection is preferred. The required amount removed (b) in a single section or (c) by progressive shaving.

cut off in a single section (Fig 8-20b) or shaved off progressively starting from the apex (Fig 8-20c). The former technique is recommended if, for example, a root apex of a maxillary tooth is in close proximity to the maxillary sinus.

Following root-end resection, the canal is uncovered and should be amenable to retrograde instrumentation and obturation, as appropriate. There is no

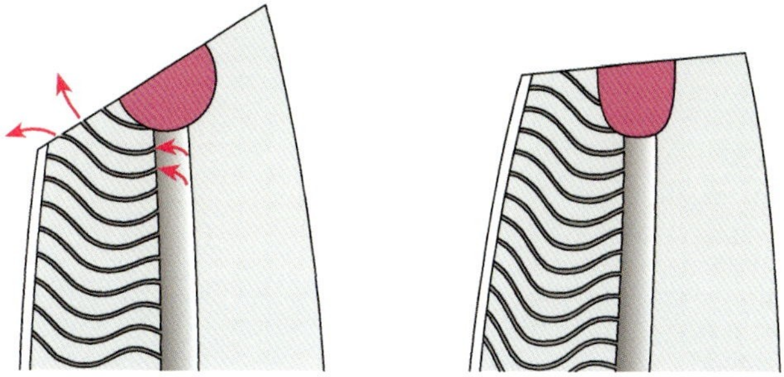

Fig 8-21 Potential pathways for leakage. (a) Exposed dentinal tubules communicating with the main canal despite a root-end filling if root face bevelled and root-end cavity prepared with a bur. (b) No such problem with a horizontal or minimally bevelled resection and an ultrasonically prepared root-end cavity.

necessity to remove an excessive amount of root, certainly not down to the base of the bony cavity.

Root-end Cavity Preparation

The need for a root-end filling has to be decided at the time of surgery when there is an opportunity to examine the seal at the cut root-end. If the root canal is filled and the seal at the cut root-end is considered adequate, there are no marginal deficiencies and no root-end filling is required (Fig 8-2). If, however, the seal is inadequate or an additional seal is considered necessary, then a root-end cavity is prepared.

In the past, root-end cavities were prepared almost exclusively with burs. There are many root-end cavity designs ranging from Class I cavities to slots. One of the disadvantages of using a bur is that the resultant cavity may not be centred on the canal and along the long axis of the root. Often, when access is limited, the cavity ends up misdirected towards (Fig 8-22a) or even perforating the palatal wall of the root. The resultant cavity may also be larger than desired and canal debris may be left on the buccal cavity wall.

Nowadays, root-end cavities are best prepared with ultrasound and specially designed, small, angled surgical ultrasonic tips (Fig 8-23). Made of stainless steel and often diamond-coated, the tips come in various shapes and sizes for easy access (Fig 8-24). Their advantages include:

- improved surgical access
- minimal to no bevelling required

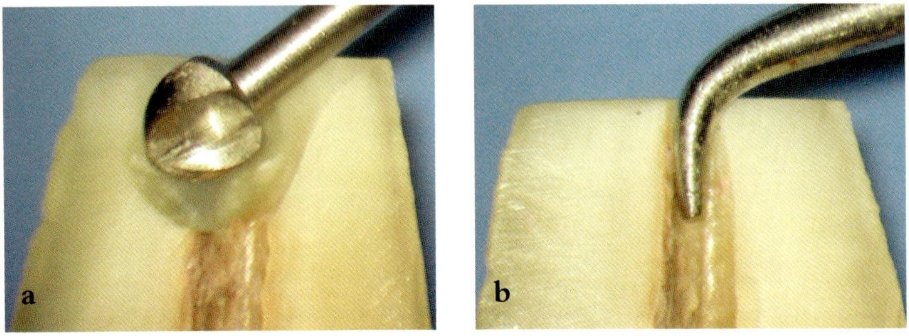

Fig 8-22 Root-end cavity preparation. (a) With a bur, the resultant cavity is often misdirected palatally. (b) Nowadays, a cavity is prepared along the long axis of the root using a microsurgical ultrasonic tip.

- cavity preparation along the long axis of the root (Fig 8-22b)
- greater depth of cavity preparation
- debridement of root-end and isthmuses
- potential removal of smear layer.

The root-end cavity should ideally be 3 mm in depth to ensure an adequate root-end filling. A 3 mm root-end resection together with 3 mm axial cavity preparation creates an optimal "apical control zone" of 6 mm (Fig 8-25).

Root-end Filling

The requirements of an ideal root-end filling material are well documented (Box 8-1). Amalgam has traditionally been used for root-end fillings, but there are a number of disadvantages with this material:

- corrosion and dimensional changes with moisture contamination
- lack of effective seal
- low success rate in clinical studies (Fig 8-26)
- introduction of mercury into the body
- unsightly amalgam tattoos from excess material (Fig 8-27).

Alternatives have therefore been sought, and well-documented evidence is available to support the use of:

Reinforced zinc oxide-eugenol cements

Zinc oxide-eugenol cements have been used as root-end filling materials for a number of years. They are now amongst the materials being promoted as substitutes for amalgam root-end fillings. Originally, zinc oxide-eugenol

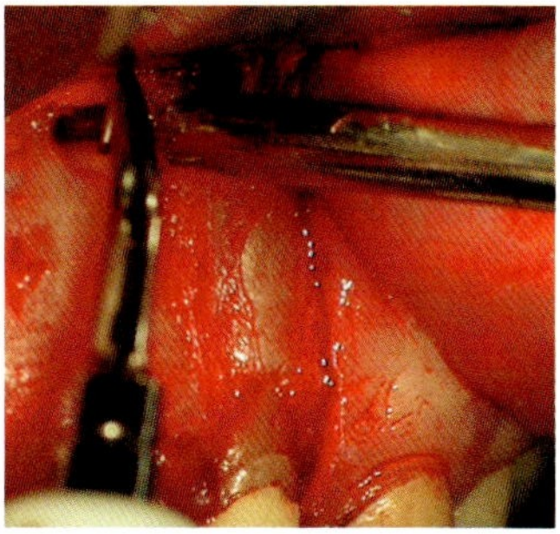

Fig 8-23 Root-end cavity preparation with a microsurgical ultrasonic tip.

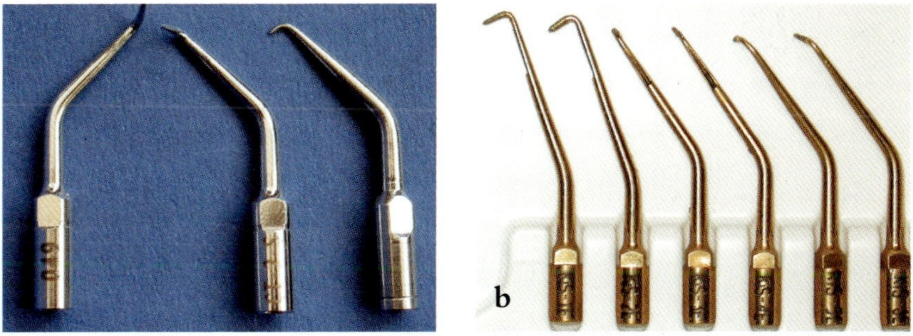

Fig 8-24 Microsurgical ultrasonic tips. (a) Stainless steel. (b) Diamond-coated.

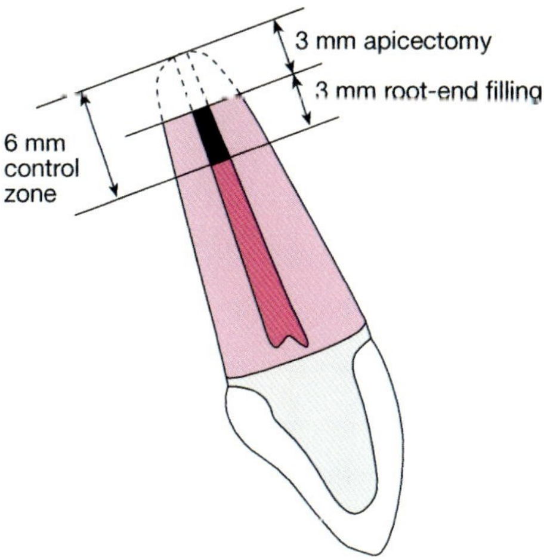

Fig 8-25 A 3 mm root-end resection plus a 3 mm axial cavity to form an "apical control zone" of 6 mm.

Box 8-1

The requirements of an ideal root-end filling material

Root-end filling materials should:

- *Adhere or bond to tooth tissue and seal the root-end three dimensionally.*
- *Not promote, and preferably inhibit, the growth of pathogenic microorganisms.*
- *Be dimensionally stable and unaffected by moisture in either the set or unset state.*
- *Be well tolerated by periapical tissues with no inflammatory reactions.*
- *Stimulate the regeneration of normal periodontium.*
- *Be non-toxic both locally and systemically.*
- *Not corrode or be electrochemically active.*
- *Not stain the tooth or the periapical tissues.*
- *Be easily distinguishable on radiographs.*
- *Have a long shelf life, be easy to mix and insert.*

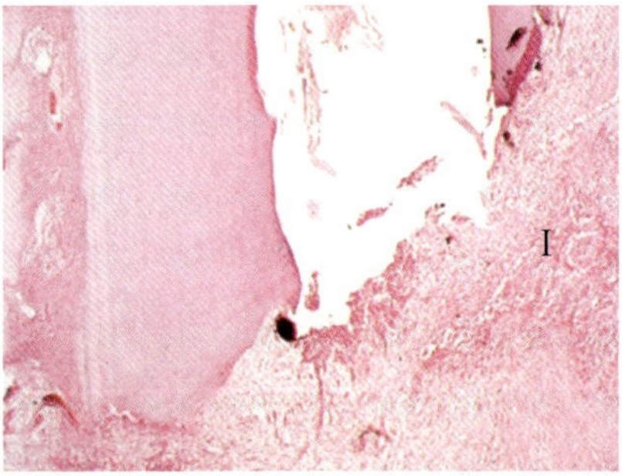

Fig 8-26 Histological section of root-end showing severe inflammation (I) adjacent to the root face where amalgam, removed during processing, was used as root-end filling. (Reproduced with permission from Chong BS, et al. 1997, Int Endo J Blackwell Publishing, Oxford.)

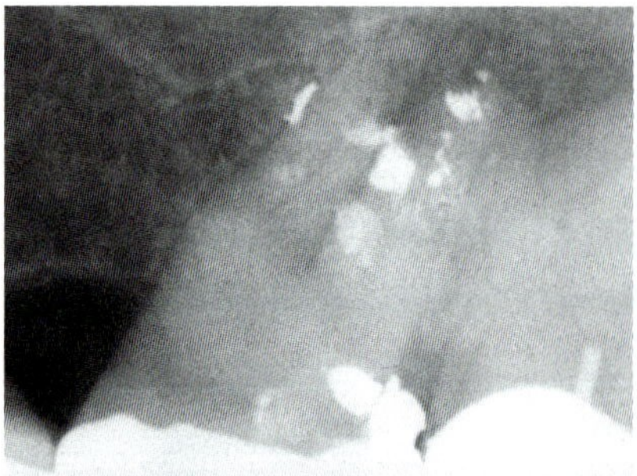

Fig 8-27 "Shotgun pellets" appearance of excess amalgam root-end filling lodged in periapical tissues may cause gingival tattooing.

cements were weak, had long setting times and were likely to be absorbed over time, but modified versions have been developed:

- Ethoxybenzoic acid (EBA) cement (Stailine Super EBA, Staident International, Staines, UK) (Fig 8-28a), improved by the partial substitution of eugenol liquid with o-ethoxybenzoic acid and the addition of fused quartz or aluminium oxide to the powder.

- Intermediate Restorative Material (IRM) (Dentsply DeTrey-DeDent, Konstanz, Germany) (Fig 8-28b), reinforced by the addition of polymethymethacrylate to the powder.

Mineral Trioxide Aggregate (MTA)

Developed in California, USA, MTA has been extensively investigated for root-end filling. The chemical composition of MTA is very similar to Portland cement. However, Portland cement is very heterogeneous and may contain impurities. In contrast, MTA is homogeneous and consistent in composition. Many root-end filling materials are not moisture-tolerant but MTA requires moisture to set. The MTA, in powder-form, consists of fine hydrophilic particles. When mixed with sterile water, hydration of the MTA results in a colloidal gel that solidifies into a hard structure. Commercially formulated MTA is marketed as ProRoot MTA (Dentsply Maillefer, Ballaigues, Switzerland) (Fig 8-29).

MTA has shown excellent sealing ability and good biocompatibility. Unlike other current root-end filling materials, hard tissue repair (cementum) has also been observed to occur directly on the surface of the material (Fig 8-30). Cementum formation is a sign of regeneration and may represent the ultimate biological seal of the root end and exposed dentinal tubules. It has been reported that MTA appears to induce cementogenesis by offering a biologically active substrate for osteoblasts, allowing good adherence of the bone cells to the material. It also stimulates cytokine production. Since MTA has a long setting time (2 hours 45 mins ± 5 mins), it must not be disturbed until fully set. Further developments are also necessary to improve the handling qualities of the material and make it easier to pack. The first prospec-

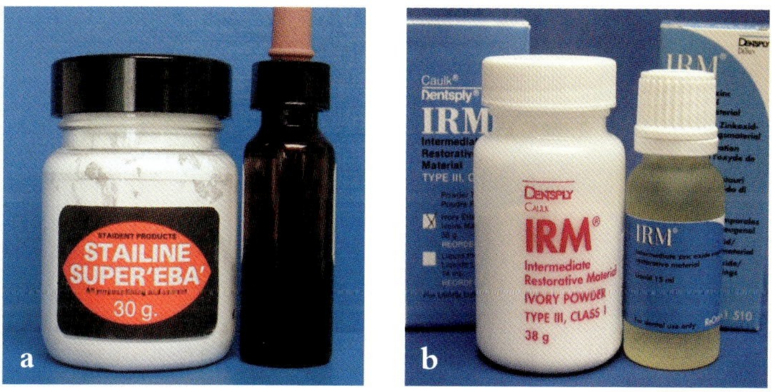

Fig 8-28 Reinforced zinc oxide-eugenol cements. (a) EBA. (b) IRM.

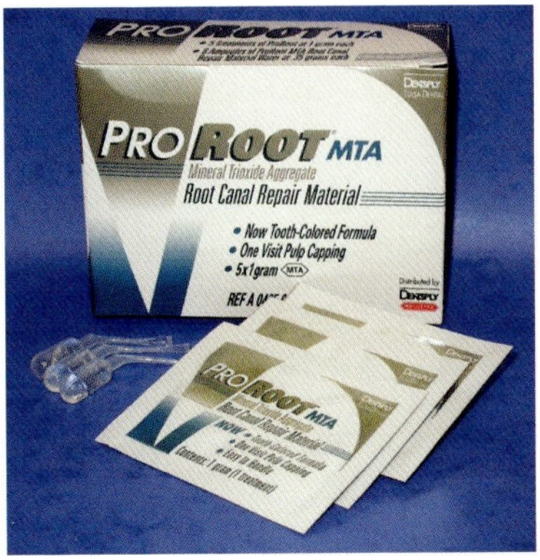

Fig 8-29 Commercially available MTA.

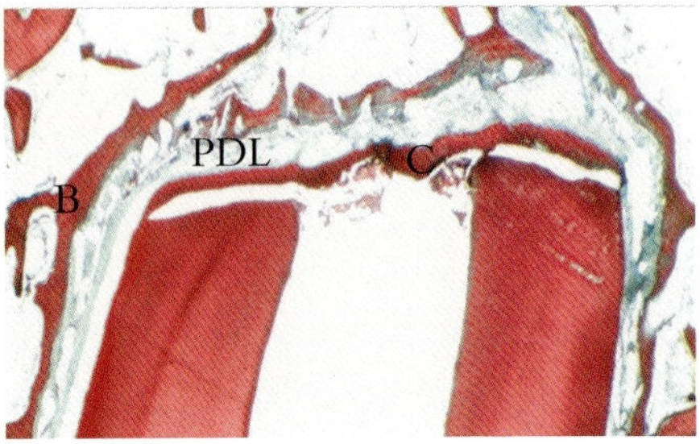

Fig 8-30 Histological section of root-end where MTA was used showing cementum (C) formation, periodontal ligament (PDL) and bone (B). MTA removed from the root-end cavity during histological processing. (Courtesy of T.R. Pitt Ford and M. Torabinejad).

tive clinical study on the use of MTA as a root-end filling material followed up to 2 years reported a high success rate although it was not significantly better than using IRM.

Whichever root-end filling material is chosen, it must be mixed according to manufacturers' directions. Before placement of the root-end filling, the bony cavity may be packed with ribbon gauze to stop blood seepage and ensure excess material is not lodged around the cut root end. If there is still bleeding on to the root end, a local haemostatic agent may be applied (Fig 8-31). A small cotton pellet moistened with local anaesthetic solution containing epinephrine (adrenaline) may be applied to the bony crypt to aid haemostasis. Epinephrine 1:1000, typically in ampoules as an emergency drug, is even more effective but should be used with caution and not left in place for more than a minute. Ferric sulphate (15–20%) solution is another effective haemostatic agent, but it is very acidic (pH 0.8–1.6) and should be used sparingly; it may also cause tattooing if not washed away completely before wound closure. There are many other haemostatic agents available including medical grade Plaster of Paris and absorbable lyophilised collagen (Hémocollagène, Spécialités Septodont, Saint-Maur, France and CollaCote, Colla-tec Inc. Plainsboro, NJ, USA). Some haemostatic agents such as bone wax (88% beeswax, 12% isopropyl palmitate) are non-absorbable, may affect healing, and are no longer recommended.

The prepared root-end cavity is dried with paper points prior to inserting the root-end filling. Alternatively, a microsurgical irrigator (Stropko irrigator,

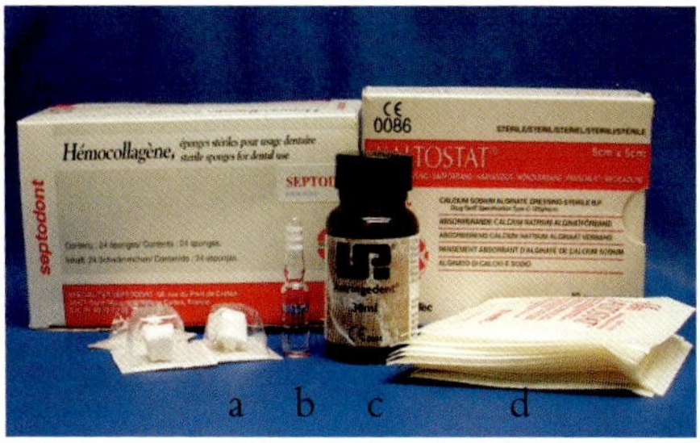

Fig 8-31 Selection of local haemostatic agents. (a) Lyophilised collagen sponges (Hémocollagène). (b) Epinephrine 1:1000 ampoule. (c) Ferric sulphate solution (Astringedent). (d) Calcium alginate dressing (Kaltostat).

SybronEndo, Orange, CA, USA) (Fig 8-32), which fits into the 3-in-1 syringe, after adjusting the water and air pressure, will allow directional microcontrol of air and water. Root-end filling carriers (Fig 8-33) including those specially designed for MTA (Dovgan MTA carriers, Quality Aspirators, Duncansville, TX, USA) (Fig 8-34) aid accurate material placement. To help improve condensation of root-end fillings, specially designed pluggers are available. Alternatively, a sickle-shaped explorer modified by flattening its tip may be used. After root-end filling, a small-bore sucker-tip (SybronEndo, Orange, CA, USA) (Fig 8-35) is used to remove surplus material. With MTA, the surface of the root filling is wiped with a damp cotton pellet to smooth the material and remove any excess. The adaptation of the root-end filling is inspected with magnifying loupes or an operating microscope and surgical micro-mirrors. These mirrors are 4–5 mm in diameter and are made of either polished stainless steel (SybronEndo, Orange, CA, USA) (Fig 8-36a) or sapphire glass (Fig 8-36b). All packing material must be removed and the surgical site washed thoroughly with saline to flush out any debris. If a slow-setting material such

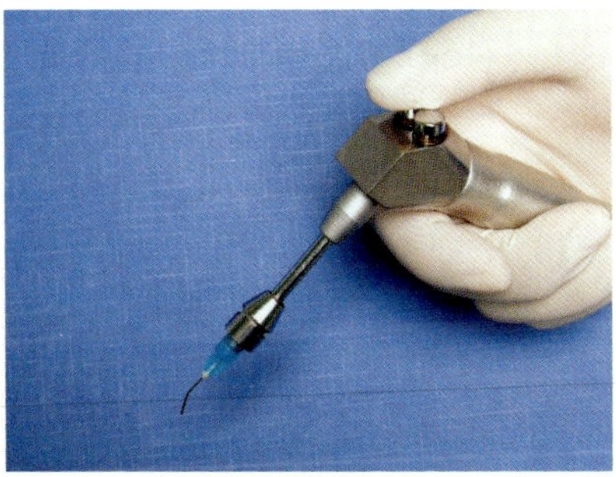

Fig 8-32 A microsurgical irrigator for drying the root-end cavity prior to filling placement.

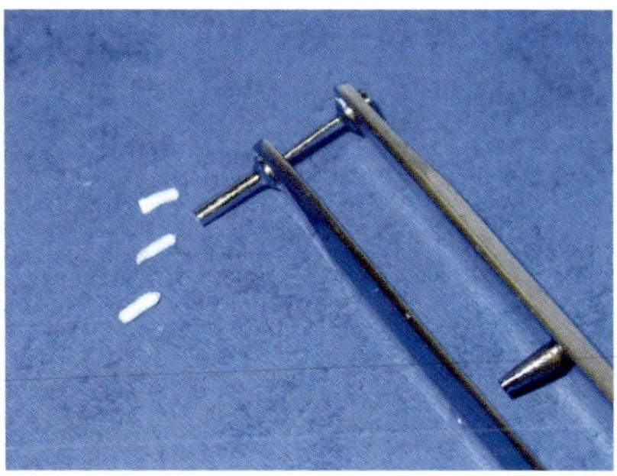

Fig 8-33 Root-end filling carrier.

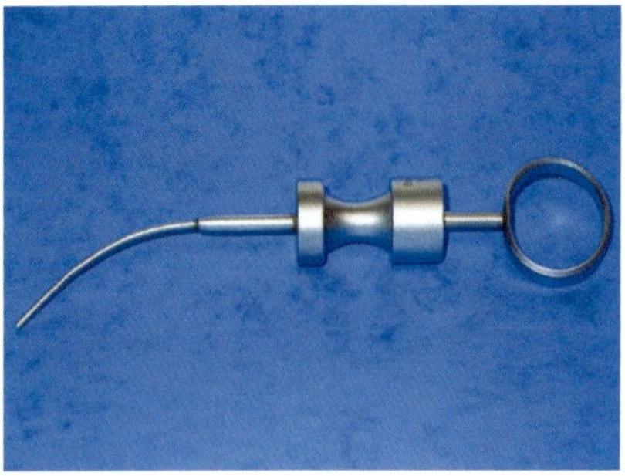

Fig 8-34 Dovgan MTA carrier.

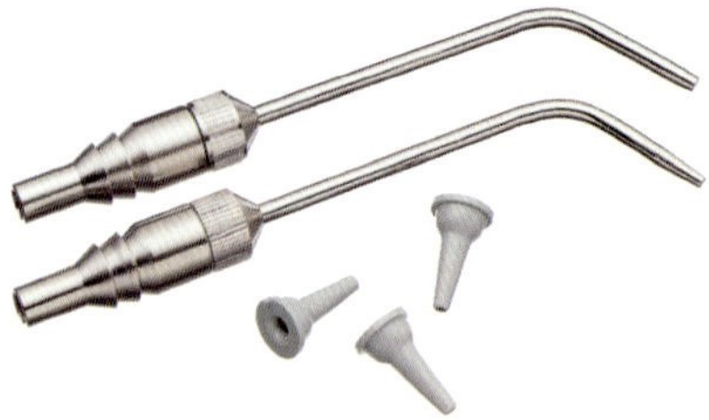

Fig 8-35 Microsurgical suction tube and rubber suction tips.

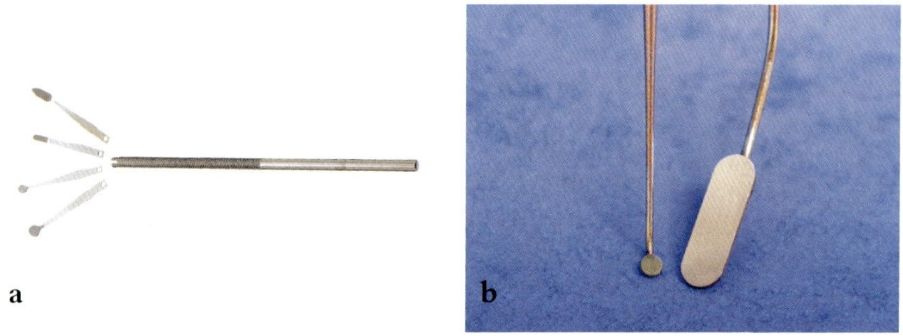

Fig 8-36 Surgical micro-mirrors. (a) Polished stainless steel. (b) Sapphire glass.

as MTA is used, debridement should be undertaken with care to avoid washing out of the root-end filling. A radiograph is then taken to check the technical quality of the procedure and for the records.

Guided Tissue Regeneration

After surgery, bony infill should occur predictably in periapical bone defects. Rapid bone regeneration can be encouraged by the use of guided tissue regeneration techniques employing:

- membranes or barriers
- bone grafts
- synthetic bone substitutes.

They may be of particular value in situations where there is:

- a large periapical lesion

- a through-and-through lesion, perforating both cortical plates
- an endodontic-periodontal lesion.

Guided tissue regeneration techniques can enhance the quality and quantity of bone reformation, but they will not alter the tissue response at the root-end. Careful case selection, experience and a meticulous technique are essential for success. Guided regeneration techniques should not be undertaken in the absence of suitable training.

Flap Replacement and Suturing

The tissue flap is gently and accurately replaced. Firm pressure is applied indirectly with a piece of saline-soaked gauze for a few minutes to help wound reapproximation and haemostasis. Sutures are placed to stabilise the reflected tissues. A minimum number of single interrupted (Fig 8-37) or sling (Fig 8-38) sutures should be placed, according to operator preference and sufficient to hold the flap in position. Too many sutures (Fig 8-39) are of no additional benefit and may delay healing. Sutures vary in gauge sizes; they may also be:

- absorbable, or non-absorbable
- monofilament or multifilament
- braided or twisted
- dyed or undyed
- coated (e.g. PTFE impregnated) or uncoated.

Multifilament, non-absorbable, braided silk sutures are popular and easier to handle than monofilament nylon or gut. However, a number of monofilament sutures (e.g. Supramid, S. Jackson Inc., Alexandria, VA, USA; Ethilon, Ethicon Ltd., Edinburgh, UK) with improved handling characteristics are also available.

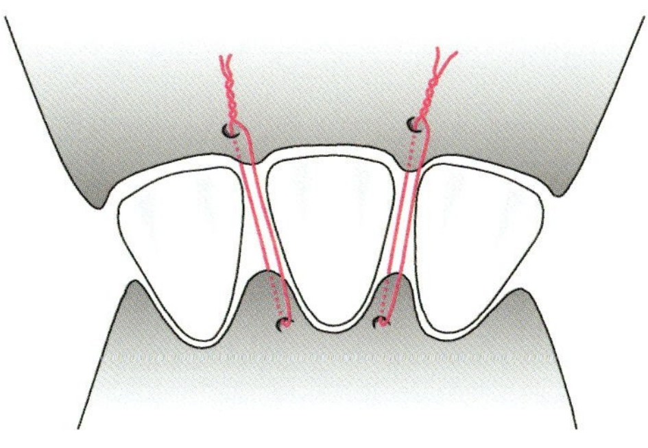

Fig 8-37 Single, interrupted sutures to reapproximate the tissue flap.

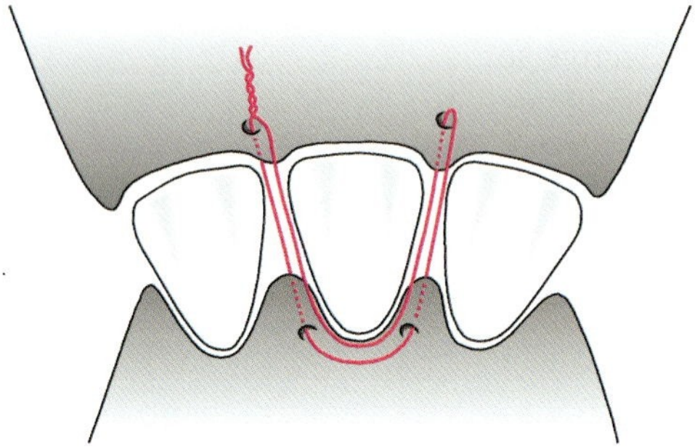

Fig 8-38 Sling suture to reapproximate the tissue flap.

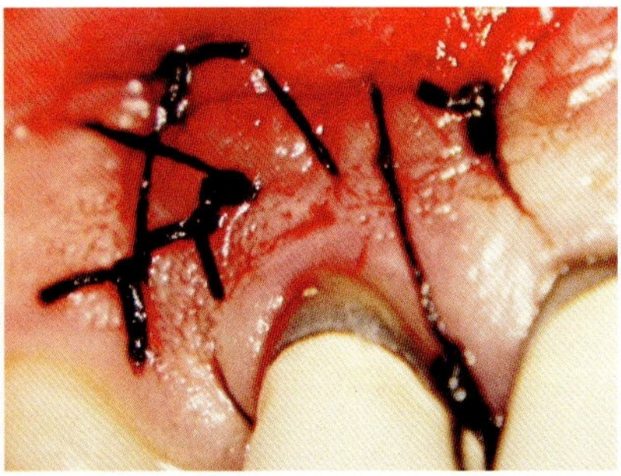

Fig 8-39 Too many sutures are not beneficial and may delay healing.

The size of the suture should allow sufficient flexibility but not be so thick as to tear the mucosa; metric size 1 or 1.5 (USP size 5-0 or 4-0) sutures are suitable. The needle is made of stainless steel and comes in varying shapes and sizes. The needle should be able to pass through the interproximal spaces without undue difficulty and puncture the tissue flap cleanly without causing damage.

After the sutures are placed, further tissue compression is carried out for a few minutes to reduce the thickness of the blood clot under the flap and encourage healing by primary intention. An ice pack (see also postoperative care) may be applied immediately, 10 minutes "on" and 5 minutes "off," to help reduce swelling.

Sutures should be removed once the wound is stabilized, as early as 48–72 hours postoperatively. They should certainly not be left longer than required as prolonged suture retention will merely delay healing.

Postoperative Care
Analgesics may be prescribed if severe pain is anticipated. Non-prescription NSAIDs are very effective so narcotic analgesics are seldom necessary for postoperative pain management. For maximum effectiveness, two different analgesics may be staggered – for example, Paracetamol (Acetaminophen) with Ibuprofen, to avoid the peaks and troughs of pain control; these two drugs also have additive analgesic effect when taken together and are well tolerated in most patients for short-term use. A new generation of selective cyclooxygenase-2 (COX-2) inhibitors (e.g. Rofecoxib) has come on the market and holds promise, with all the therapeutic effects but not the adverse effects associated with traditional, non-selective NSAIDs.

Antibiotics are seldom necessary as post-surgical infection is rare. If indicated, the choice of antibiotics and regime should be similar to that for treating an acute dental infection.

The patient should be given both oral and written instructions on postoperative care. These should include the following:

- **Do not** eat, drink or rinse your mouth for 2 hours after surgery.
- **Wound** should not be disturbed for the first 24 hours. The wound is stitched and it is best not to lift the lip to examine the incision as this may dislodge the sutures (stitches). The sutures are removed 3–7 days after the operation and an appointment for this should have been arranged.
- **Swelling** may occur some hours after surgery and may be delayed by 24 hours. To reduce this swelling, apply an ice pack (crushed ice in a plastic bag or a bag of frozen peas, wrapped in a towel) to the face (20 minutes in every hour) and repeat several times during the day of surgery.
- **Bruising** is a relatively rare occurrence but when it does occur it can be extensive and can take some days to disappear.
- **Pain** is not a major feature of apicectomy but there is, inevitably, a certain amount of postoperative discomfort, which is easily controlled by taking commonly available, non-prescription painkillers/analgesics such as Paracetamol and Codeine or Ibuprofen. Aspirin is best avoided as it will interfere with blood clotting. Ensure that any analgesic taken is well tolerated, without any adverse effects and not incompatible with other routine medications prescribed. The analgesic should be taken on a regular basis, every 4–6 hourly, starting one hour after the procedure. Analgesics work much better if taken before the onset of pain/discomfort.
- **Oral hygiene** should be maintained. Teeth away from the operation site may be brushed normally, possibly more carefully than usual. The operation site should be kept clean with mouthwashes, in particular after

eating. A mouthwash of chlorhexidine gluconate 0.2% (Fig 8-7) may also be used. An alternative mouthwash may be made by adding half a tablespoon of salt to a tumbler of warm water. Mouthwashes should be continued until healing is complete or at least until the sutures are removed.

- **Eating, drinking, alcohol and smoking**, there are no absolute restrictions on these, but common sense should prevail and food chosen should be soft and easily chewed. Alcohol and smoking should be avoided to improve healing.
- **Medication**, like antibiotics and painkillers/analgesics, if prescribed, should be taken as instructed.
- **Strenuous exercise** should be avoided for at least one day after the operation.

Patient Review

At the suture removal appointment, healing should be checked. The incisional wound healing process can be briefly divided into the following stages:

- clotting and inflammation
- epithelial healing
- connective tissue healing
- maturation and remodelling.

After suture removal, provided healing is uneventful, a new appointment should be made to review the patient in 6–12 months' time when a radiograph should be taken to monitor healing. Scarring may be visible initially but, with time, the scars will mature and become less visible. Usually, osseous healing is evident radiographically and often complete after one year; combined with evidence of clinical healing, further follow-up may be unnecessary. Otherwise, further follow-up for up to four years, as prescribed by ESE guidelines (see Chapter 1), is essential to determine treatment outcome.

Conclusions

- Apicectomy and root-end filling is indicated if non-surgical retreatment is unsuccessful or impracticable, and as an adjunct to non-surgical retreatment.
- The presence of a good-quality root filling is crucial to the successful outcome of surgery.
- The root apex should be apicected horizontally and not bevelled more than necessary to allow good vision.
- If the root canal is already filled, a root-end filling is not always required provided the seal at the apex is considered adequate.

- Ultrasonic root-end cavity preparation has many advantages over the use of burs.
- Amalgam is no longer considered the root-end filling of choice. Reinforced zinc oxide-eugenol cements and MTA have emerged as popular and more effective alternatives to amalgam.

Further Reading

Carr GB. Ultrasonics root end preparation. Dent Clinics N Am 1997;41:541-554.

Chong BS. MTA – many tested applications. Dentistry 2001;2:18-20.

Chong BS, Pitt Ford TR, Hudson MB. A prospective clinical study of Mineral Trioxide Aggregate and IRM when used as root-end filling materials in endodontic surgery. Int Endod J 2003;36:520-526.

Chong BS, Ford TR, Kariyawasam SP. Tissue response to potential root-end filling materials in infected root canals. Int Endod J 1997;30:102-114.

Danin J, Linder LE, Lundqvist G, et al. Outcomes of periradicular surgery in cases with apical pathosis and untreated canals. Oral Surg Oral Med Oral Pathol Oral Radiol Endod 1999;87:227-232.

Lin LM, Gaengler P, Langeland K. Periradicular curettage. Int Endod J 1996;29:220-227.

Pecora G, Baek S-H, Rethman S, Kim S. Barrier membrane techniques in endodontic microsurgery. Dent Clinics N Am 1997;41:585-602.

Velvart P. Papilla base incision: a new approach to recession-free healing of the interdental papilla after endodontic surgery. Int Endod J 2002;35:453-460.

Witherspoon DE, Gutmann JL. Haemostasis in periradicular surgery. Int Endod J 1996;29:135-149.

Index

Quintessentials for General Dental Practitioners Series

in 36 volumes

Editor-in-Chief: Professor Nairn H F Wilson

The Quintessentials for General Dental Practitioners Series covers basic principles and key issues in all aspects of modern dental medicine. Each book can be read as a stand-alone volume or in conjunction with other books in the series.

	Publication date, approximately
Oral Surgery and Oral Medicine, Editor: John G Meechan	
Practical Dental Local Anaesthesia	available
Practical Oral Medicine	Autumn 2004
Practical Conscious Sedation	available
Practical Surgical Dentistry	Autumn 2004
Imaging, Editor: Keith Horner	
Interpreting Dental Radiographs	available
Panoramic Radiology	Autumn 2004
Twenty-first Century Dental Imaging	Autumn 2004
Periodontology, Editor: Iain L C Chapple	
Understanding Periodontal Diseases: Assessment and Diagnostic Procedures in Practice	available
Decision-Making for the Periodontal Team	available
Successful Periodontal Therapy – A Non-Surgical Approach	available
Periodontal Management of Children, Adolescents and Young Adults	available
Periodontal Medicine: A Window on the Body	Autumn 2005
Implantology, Editor: Lloyd J Searson	
Implantology in General Dental Practice	Autumn 2004
Managing Orofacial Pain in Practice	Summer 2005

750.364 LARCENY; FROM LIBRARIES

SEC. 364. LARCENY FROM LIBRARIES - - ANY PERSON WHO SHALL PROCURE, OR TAKE IN ANY WAY FROM ANY PUBLIC LIBRARY OR THE LIBRARY OF ANY LITERARY, SCIENTIFIC, HISTORICAL OR LIBRARY SOCIETY OR ASSOCIATION, WHETHER INCORPORATED OR UNINCORPORATED, ANY BOOK, PAMPHLET, MAP, CHART, PAINTING, PICTURE, PHOTOGRAPH, PERIODICAL, NEWSPAPER, MAGAZINE, MANUSCRIPT OR EXHIBIT OR ANY PART THEREOF, WITH INTENT TO CONVERT THE SAME TO HIS OWN USE, OR WITH INTENT TO DEFRAUD THE OWNER THEREOF, OR WHO HAVING PROCURED OR TAKEN ANY SUCH BOOK, PAMPHLET, MAP, CHART, PAINTING, PICTURE, PHOTOGRAPH, PERIODICAL, NEWSPAPER, MAGAZINE, MANUSCRIPT OR EXHIBIT OR ANY PART THEREOF, SHALL THEREAFTER CONVERT THE SAME TO HIS OWN USE OR FRAUDULENTLY DEPRIVE THE OWNER THEREOF, SHALL BE GUILTY OF A MISDEMEANOR.

MICHIGAN COMPILED LAWS.